T0206708

"This is a story that simply had to be [...] conviction and of leadership which ha[...] less lives since the early 1970s ... Being raised in Melbourne I recall when the road toll was 1034 and how that became the public tipping point for all the action that has followed and which is so well chronicled in this most valuable book."

Professor Chris Baggoley
Australian Chief Medical Officer 2011–2016

"In implementing regional trauma networks across England, I was truly indebted to the work done in Victoria and the lessons learned. I am sure I will not be alone in recognising the enormous contribution the Victorian State Trauma System has made to the improvement of trauma care worldwide."

Professor Keith Willett
Director for Acute Care, NHS England

"This is a remarkable public health success story for the world, about how a health systems approach could potentially save millions of lives."

Dr Nobhojit Roy
National Health Systems Resource Centre Advisor,
Ministry of Health & Family Welfare, Government of India

"The Victorian State Trauma System is a model for comprehensive trauma care. Lessons learned from the development of this system should be applicable across the globe."

Professor Eileen Bulger
Chair, American College of Surgeons Committee on Trauma

"Victoria has demonstrated that scientific use of local data can drive system change and deliver world leading clinical outcomes."

Professor Ian Civil
Clinical Leader, New Zealand Major Trauma National Clinical Network

"Victoria has pioneered the assessment of long term outcomes after injury and sparked global initiatives to reduce trauma-related disability."

Professor Avery Nathens
Chair, Ontario Trauma Advisory Committee, Toronto, Canada; and
Director, American College of Surgeons Trauma Quality Improvement Program

"The Victorian State Trauma System has shown the way forward for the epidemic of trauma – reducing mortality and adding productive years of life."

Professor Mahesh Misra
former Director, All India Institute of Medical Sciences, Delhi, India

"After studying the Victorian approach I was able to successfully reduce preventable trauma deaths at Khon Kaen Regional Hospital year upon year."

Dr Witaya Chadbunchachai
Director, WHO Collaborating Centre for Injury Prevention and Safety Promotion,
Khon Kaen, Thailand

"As a leading cause of death globally, all countries must do what they can to prevent injury and build and maintain a 'chain of survival' for those who do get injured. The Victorian State Trauma System is a superb example of a locally-developed comprehensive system of prevention, prehospital care, hospital-based care, and rehabilitation, with high quality data to demonstrate its effect on outcomes. The effort made by the authors to describe its development and implementation is admirable, and should help others to follow Victoria's lead."

Dr Tina Gaarder
President, International Association for Trauma Surgery and Intensive Care

From Roadside to Recovery

FROM ROADSIDE TO RECOVERY

The Story of the Victorian State Trauma System

Peter Bragge

Associate Professor and Director of Health Programs, BehaviourWorks Australia,
Monash Sustainable Development Institute, Monash University,
Melbourne, Australia

Russell Gruen

Professor and Dean, College of Health and Medicine,
Australian National University,
Canberra, Australia

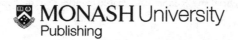
MONASH University Publishing

From Roadside to Recovery: The Story of the Victorian State Trauma System

Monash University Publishing
Matheson Library and Information Services Building
40 Exhibition Walk
Monash University
Clayton, Victoria 3800, Australia
www.publishing.monash.edu

ISBN: 9781925495799 (paperback)
ISBN: 9781925495805 (pdf)
ISBN: 9781925495812 (epub)

www.publishing.monash.edu/books/frr-9781925495799.html

Series: Monash Studies in Australian Society

Design: Les Thomas

Cover image: Front page of *The Sun News Pictorial* on November 24, 1970. An attempt to represent the 1969 road toll of 1034 using schoolchildren in the main street of Red Cliffs, near Mildura. The organisers had wanted 1034 to lie down, but ran out of children at 975. Image used with permission of News Corp Australia and subject to copyright.

This project has proudly been supported by TAC.

A catalogue record for this book is available from the National Library of Australia

Printed in Australia by Griffin Press an Accredited ISO AS/NZS 14001:2004 Environmental Management System printer.

FSC
www.fsc.org
MIX
Paper from responsible sources
FSC® C009448

The paper this book is printed on is certified against the Forest Stewardship Council ® Standards. Griffin Press holds FSC chain of custody certification SGS-COC-005088. FSC promotes environmentally responsible, socially beneficial and economically viable management of the world's forests.

CONTENTS

ACKNOWLEDGEMENTS

The authors gratefully acknowledge:

The Victorian Transport Accident Commission for their support of this work;

News Corp Australia in granting permission to republish images and articles in this book. All images and articles are subject to copyright;

Coretext editor Brad Collis, writer Bianca Nogrady and in particular writer Melissa Marino who produced most of the profiles featured throughout the chapters;

Participants in the 2011 conference "From Roadside to Recovery," who provided inspiration and material for the book;

All those who agreed to participate in or contribute to the profiles featured in the book; and especially Micaela Henderson, who gave her first-person account of experiencing the Victorian State Trauma System as a patient;

Our partners, Michelle and Theresa, and children, Emily, Lucas, Spencer and Kody, who have supported us to be able to tell this story.

ABOUT THE AUTHORS

Peter Bragge PhD, B. Physio (Hons.), L.T.C.L.

Peter Bragge is an Associate Professor in healthcare behaviour change at BehaviourWorks Australia (BWA), part of the Monash Sustainable Development Institute. As Director of BWA's Health Programs, he works closely with government and industry partners to define, understand and address high-priority healthcare challenges using a range of strategies informed by behaviour change theory and research evidence.

He has led projects for numerous government agencies including The Victorian Department of Health and Human Services, Victorian Department of Premier and Cabinet, Victorian Transport Accident Commission, Victorian Managed Insurance Authority, WorkSafe Victoria and The NSW Environment Protection Authority. He also collaborates with international researchers in the fields of trauma care and behavioural science across Canada, Europe, and the USA.

He has published over 50 articles in academic journals including *The Lancet* and is also active in popular science media such as *The Conversation*. Peter currently serves on the board of the Spinal Cord Injury Network and provides expert advice across a range of other committees and clinical areas.

Prior to his research career, Peter worked for 10 years as a physiotherapist in public and private practice settings, including one year in the United Kingdom. His physiotherapy career included senior roles in the intensive care and inpatient physiotherapy management of acute spinal cord injury, often as a result of road trauma. This work, combined with his long-term involvement with research funded by the Victorian Transport Accident Commission, inspired him in writing this book.

Peter is also a keen musician with a background in classical piano. He plays in a jazz and grooves band with regular gigs around Melbourne, where he lives with his wife Michelle and their two children, Emily and Lucas.

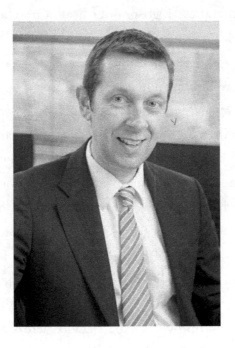

Russell L. Gruen MBBS PhD FRACS

Russell Gruen is a pioneer in surgery and health systems research. From 2006 to 2015 he was a consultant trauma surgeon at The Royal Melbourne Hospital and then The Alfred Hospital – Victoria's two designated adult Major Trauma Services, where he cared for the State's most severely injured people. From 2009 to 2015 he was also Professor of Surgery and Public Health at Monash University, and Director of the National Trauma Research Institute.

Having trained in Victoria's metropolitan and rural hospitals, he received his medical degree from the University of Melbourne and his Fellowship in General Surgery from the Royal Australasian College of Surgeons, after which he undertook specialist trauma surgery training in Seattle, USA. He also completed a PhD through Flinders University on access to surgical care for remote Aboriginal people in northern Australia, and then a Harkness Fellowship in Healthcare Policy, a Fellowship in Medical Ethics, and the Advanced Management Program, all at Harvard. He led development of the Australian Trauma Registry and the Australia-India Trauma Systems Collaboration, and he was a founding member of the WHO Global Alliance for Care of the Injured, and a Lancet Commissioner in Global Surgery.

In 2015 he moved to Singapore with his wife, Theresa, and sons Spencer and Kody. Russell was the founding Professor of Surgery at the Lee Kong Chian School of Medicine and Tan Tock Seng Hospital, and Executive Director of the NTU Institute for Health Technologies at Nanyang Technological University. In 2019 he will return to Australia as Dean of the College of Health and Medicine at the Australian National University, and a surgeon at The Canberra Hospital.

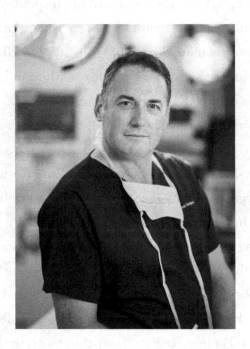

PROLOGUE

By Melissa Marino

Micaela Henderson has no recollection of the 2010 car crash that nearly killed her, but she knows the night started like many others before it.

A summer's evening, an outdoor party beckoning and, as is common for young people socialising in country Victoria, the obligatory drive to the destination. There was nothing remarkable about it. Not a hint that anything could go wrong.

But on the way to the Harrow B&S (Bachelors and Spinsters) Ball – typical of many held regularly around rural Australia – everything for the 23 year old agricultural science student and farmhand changed. The car in which Micaela was a passenger hit a patch of gravel on the road and, through no fault of the driver, veered out of control and slammed into a tree at 100 kilometres an hour.

Micaela, thrown some distance from the car, was found by a farmer who, alerted by the screams of the trapped driver, chanced upon the crash as he was checking stock water on his remote property.

Micaela lay silent.

Unconscious, and with a massive head injury, her broken and bloodied body was tangled in a barbed wire fence. The farmer immediately phoned the Triple-0 emergency number on his mobile phone, while Micaela remained motionless.

Soon after, an ambulance helicopter landed.

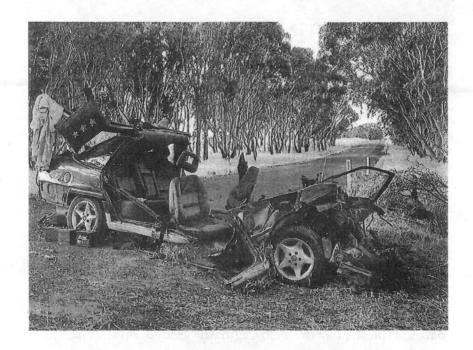

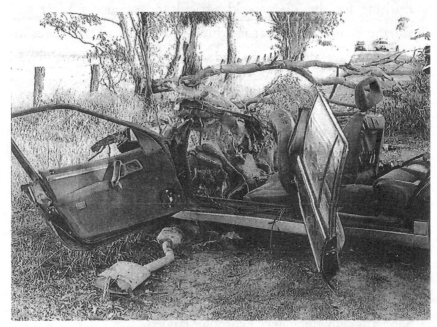

Photo from the scene of Micaela's car crash, January 2010

Image supplied by Victoria Police under Freedom of information

Had this crash happened 20 years earlier Micaela would almost certainly have died. But in 2010, a revolutionary world class trauma response system kicked into gear and – with her own tenacious spirit – she has lived to tell her story; a personal experience that embodies more than three decades of dedicated work by doctors, politicians, community leaders and campaigning journalists to develop a whole new way of responding to trauma, especially road trauma, that puts people ahead of institutions and, more importantly, ahead of blame and money.

What you are about to read in this book is the story of a comprehensive emergency, medical, education, and insurance system put into place to drive down the road toll, put a stop to preventable

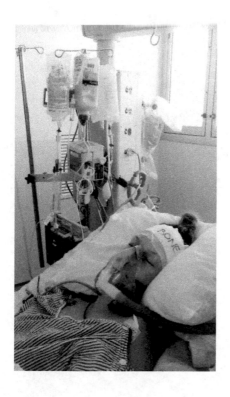

Micaela Henderson after having brain surgery following her car crash, January 2010
Image supplied by Micaela Henderson, taken by Marie Henderson

deaths, reduce disabling injuries and help survivors, like Micaela, to recover and get a second chance at life.

It's a system integral to the future Micaela now has in front of her. Micaela's story, which we will return to at the end of the book, is the story of the Victorian State Trauma System, the VSTS.

PREFACE

By Charlie Mock

Professor of Surgery and Epidemiology, University of Washington, Seattle, USA;
Former President, International Association of Trauma Surgery and Intensive Care

Injury (such as from road traffic crashes, violence, and other causes) is a leading cause of death, disability, suffering, and economic loss around the world. Rates of death from injury rose in today's high-income countries with the advent of industrialisation and motorisation in the twentieth century. Responses to this problem were so slow that injury was termed "The neglected disease of modern society." Similarly, a wave of deaths from motor vehicle crashes is hitting today's low- and middle-income countries.

Much can be done to lower the rates of death from injury, through road safety and other forms of injury prevention, and through improvements in care of the injured (trauma care). In treatment after injury, minutes and even seconds count. Much needs to be done quickly to save life or limb. Outcomes depends on having well-trained professionals making quick decisions and having access to the tools that they need at the time they need them. Better organisation and delivery of trauma care, both outside and inside hospitals, allows such care to happen.

Better organisation of care requires outcomes to be followed carefully and patterns and trends to be understood. Better organisation of care needs to happen at hospitals and ambulance services city-wide, province-wide, and even nationwide. Promoting such systematic improvements is challenging, and the need for improvement is often not immediately apparent and the benefits can seem far off. Hence, it is very useful to have good examples of when such improvements have been made, especially at the level of large geographic areas. For this reason alone, the Victorian State Trauma System is an extremely important example from which the world can learn.

However the Victorian State Trauma System is also exemplary in other ways. First, it addresses the entire spectrum of care from prehospital, through hospital and long-term rehabilitation. Second, it comprehensively addresses the many components of care, such as training, staffing, and availability of equipment and supplies. Third, it monitors and documents the outcomes of care with a state-wide registry, providing solid data to enable effective decision-making. This registry is especially notable in that it contains not only data on survival, but also non-mortality outcomes. Fourth, the Victorian system has produced impressive results, in the form of steady decreases in the mortality rate for injured people in the entire state. Finally, all of this important work has been accomplished with only a modest price tag, the improvements in organisation and planning costing a small percentage of the care itself. These factors make the Victorian State Trauma System an example for countries around the world to follow. Its affordability makes these improvements relevant no matter what a country's economic resources.

I'm sure readers will enjoy reading about these great achievements, and I hope they will consider their relevance to trauma care and public policy in their own settings.

INTRODUCTION

In November 2011, at a hotel overlooking Melbourne's Port Philip Bay, more than 200 doctors, nurses, paramedics, politicians and managers gathered for a conference entitled "From Roadside to Recovery," hosted by the National Trauma Research Institute (NTRI). They were joined by a small number of survivors of road trauma. It was, in part, a celebration of achievement. Not only had the state of Victoria registered a decline in number of fatalities on its roads from a high of 1077 in 1970 to 288 in 2010, a six-fold decrease per capita, but recently released data had shown that the likelihood of dying once someone had been injured, everything else being equal, had more than halved in the decade since the rollout of a new statewide system of care.

A six-fold reduction in road deaths was remarkable, and testament to four decades of efforts to prevent injury through safer roads, better designed vehicles, and improved driver behaviour. A few other countries had enjoyed similar successes and, only a few months earlier in May 2011, responding to the global epidemic of road-fatalities and noting what had proved possible, the United Nations General Assembly had enshrined these strategies as pillars in a Decade of Action for Road Safety.

While the effect of injury prevention campaigns was remarkable, halving the likelihood of dying after injury was truly extraordinary. Rarely in the history of medicine had there been an intervention so effective at saving lives. That it had done so in just ten years earned the Victorian State Trauma System the reputation of being 'penicillin-esque.'

While there certainly was celebration, the conference had another purpose. The NTRI, a joint initiative of The Alfred Hospital and Monash University, was established to improve care of the injured, everywhere. It was home to the Australian Trauma Quality Improvement Program, brokered an Australia-India Trauma Systems Collaboration, and contributed to the formation of the other international trauma care alliances. In all these initiatives it was recognised that Victoria's success lit a path for other jurisdictions to follow. So, what was it that could be learned from Victoria?

What unfolded over three days, through the personal accounts and discussion among many who were central to the system's establishment, proved an incredible story. On the face of it, the Victorian State Trauma System (VSTS) was a highly coordinated and integrated system of care designed to meet every patient's critical needs - an important but hardly revolutionary underpinning. What it did that was different, and that this was even possible, however, was the product of fierce determination, public spiritedness, wisdom and experience, as well as a healthy dose of good luck. The story provides vivid real-world lessons for public policy makers, health system leaders, strategists, marketers, insurers and citizens. In fact, they are lessons for anyone who wants to make a difference. We felt compelled to retell this story and make available these lessons, which are the purposes of this book.

Of course, the system is more complex than it sounds. Serious injuries occur anywhere and at any time, and the system needed to respond accordingly, irrespective of whether a crash was on an urban street or a deserted country road. Each patient had to receive the care he or she needed in the shortest possible time. Some of this involved improving care at the roadside and in transit, some involved strengthening hospital-based reception and resuscitation, and much required rapid and effective decision-making tailored to each patient's situation. Certainly there were patients whose injuries were unsurvivable, but the system aimed to save every patient that it could. It reminds us of a fine watch – multiple interdependent moving parts working in perfect harmony. The systems of checks and balances, audit, case review and continuous quality improvement involved many organisations, committees, communications, protocols and procedures making it a worthy case study in operational excellence in austere environments.

Anyone who has worked in or lobbied government knows how difficult it can be to make even small changes to public services. Compared to what it replaced, the VSTS was neither small nor uncomplicated, it involved significant change across several sectors and organisations, and it was expensive, at least in the up-front patient care that it underwrote. It taxed motorists and it challenged civil liberties, cultural norms, professionals' income and, most of all, it challenged the status quo. Yet even in the face of stiff opposition, there are many, without whom the system would not exist today, who had refused to accept the carnage occurring on the state's roads. In telling this story, we could not give all these heroes and heroines the prominence they deserved, but we have profiled just a few – to illustrate how contingent the system was on particular individual contributions, and to chronicle how people from different walks of life took up opportunities to rally around a worthwhile cause to which they could dedicate their talents.

Significant policy and societal changes always require some special champions. But the VSTS required more. Victoria had achieved what many others in developed and developing countries had not. For the VSTS to work, the policies and activities of several government sectors and non-government agencies had to be reorganised and realigned, and incentives and enablers created so that they were all playing their part, in a coordinated fashion, to reduce the toll of road deaths and serious injuries in Victoria. Its inception in 2001 was like the moment an orchestra stops the noisy mayhem as each player tunes up, they check their tune in unison, and then launch into a delightful symphony. How did this this moment arrive for the VSTS?

At the conference it became apparent that by 2000 at least four conditions were present that created fertile ground and a unique opportunity to radically change trauma care in Victoria. Each was an achievement in itself, and perhaps together they were necessary pre-conditions for healthcare transformation on this scale in a relatively wealthy Westminster democracy.

The first was that Victorians didn't need much convincing that injury was a public policy problem, and that there was a need for action. Sparked by a 1970 campaign acknowledged as one of the most impactful of the 20th century, generations of Victorians had over the ensuing 30 years been exposed to increasingly sophisticated versions of 'it could be you' type media campaigns portraying graphic images and provocative slogans on roadside billboards, at major sporting events, and on television in their living rooms. This public awareness was allied to world-first legislative enforcement measures — compulsory wearing of seatbelts; blood alcohol and drug testing of drivers; speed limit restrictions and so on — with meaningful penalties for breaches of these laws including cancellation of driving licenses and confiscation of vehicles. And while fatalities had been declining for many years thanks to many successful road safety initiatives, daily comparisons of this year's statistics with the same time last year aroused the competitive spirit of a generally sports-obsessed public. This seemed in stark contrast to many countries where road injury was so common that people often stepped over victims without stopping to offer assistance. Victorians clearly expected government would do what it could to reduce road trauma and provide optimal care, even if it came with other types of discomfort.

The second condition was the existence of a payment system that could finance the change. Trauma care can be expensive, and it demands immediacy without knowing whether a patient can afford it or is covered by insurance. It's unfathomable to Victorians that a comatose and bleeding patient would not be rushed to hospital by an ambulance or could be turned away because of payment issues, yet that is what happens in many countries. Even trauma centres in some developed countries have had to close their doors because they admitted too many patients who lacked any means to pay for the care they needed. Interest in social insurance and application of tort law in the 1970s culminated in the legislation of a successful and sustainable compulsory third party motor accident insurance scheme the following decade, administered by the government-operated Transport Accident Commission. This scheme, still in operation over 30 years later, provided coverage of current and projected claims well into the future. Through prudent financial management, not only could direct care costs to individuals be met, but investments could be made in capital, equipment, training, research and other systemic improvements to trauma care. Debate was therefore not so vociferous about the opportunity costs of providing the healthcare needs of those seen by some sectors of the community to be mostly risk-taking young men who had brought their injuries upon themselves.

The third was an imperative for change to happen, which came in the form of 'preventable deaths.' The road toll was certainly portrayed as a tragedy, and one that could be lessened if not avoided altogether. Yet a sense of inevitability persisted through the latter part of the 20th century that bad things would always happen, and there would always be the unlucky who found themselves in harm's way. What the community couldn't stomach, however, was the idea that deaths were occurring after people had been seriously injured because the medical care they received was substandard. No one – neither the public, the medical profession, nor the politicians – liked the idea of people dying avoidable deaths. Measuring and reporting of unchanging preventable and potentially preventable death rates over a decade came to a climax with headlines in Victoria's major newspapers and lobbying by the medical profession that galvanised public opinion and demanded a political response.

And the fourth was an environment in which an effective response was possible. In Victoria, like in other democratic systems of government, progress on worthwhile issues is often stymied when they are politicised and become part of the political battlefield. Injury prevention and trauma care initiatives have at times been controversial, but through both design and good fortune they have enjoyed, and continue to enjoy, bipartisan political support since the late 1960s. This bipartisan support delivered the legislative reforms of the 1970s and 1980s. In 1999, although the public was sensitised, financing was possible, and preventable deaths were unpalatable, bipartisanship was critical due to a change in government at the very time the new trauma system was on the cusp of being legislated. That an incoming Victorian Health Minister delivered this legislation as almost his first act in office was testament to the actors who mobilised their organisations and departments to optimise the credibility and unity of their message, ensured that both sides of politics heard the many stakeholders singing the same tune, and who themselves played critical roles in the process. Several participants described the Ministerial Committee convened in 1999 to review trauma and emergency services as the most effective committee they'd ever experienced.

A fifth condition has been necessary for sustainability of the VSTS – that is, absolute commitment to monitoring and improving system performance through a next-generation data registry, robust governance, forums and protocols for reporting, deliberation and making recommendations to the Minister, and an ability to respond to emerging issues and shifting priorities. As preventable mortality declined, the human and financial costs of long term care of survivors of severe injury became more apparent, especially of those with traumatic brain or spinal cord injuries. Over time the focus has shifted from injury prevention, to saving lives, and now to optimising recovery. In many ways, the shift from prehospital and emergency department reception and resuscitation to long-term post-acute rehabilitation and community care has been as transformative as bringing in the system in the first place. The system has remained vibrant, agile, pre-emptive and exciting to this day.

While this book focuses on road trauma, about half of patients seen by the state's trauma services have sustained non-traffic related injuries, such as falls, violence, sporting or workplace injuries. However, it is road-trauma that has driven, financed and made possible the

VSTS. Without this singular focus and all the initiatives described in this book, Victoria's world-leading trauma system would probably not have evolved.

There are important aspects of road-transport injury control that are barely touched on in this story. VicRoads, responsible for licensing, vehicle registration and road infrastructure, has made great strides as a leader in safety systems for all road users, and has launched many initiatives of which crash barriers, lane dividers, traffic cameras, speed limits and safe railway level crossings are just a few. Vehicle manufacturers have also dramatically improved safety features, including technologies such as airbags, electronic stability control, forward collision warning, auto-emergency and antilock braking systems, intelligent speed and lane-keeping assistance, driver attention detection, blind-spot warning systems, reversing cameras, seatbelt pre-tensioners, and tyre pressure monitors. All of these things have made driving much safer, and enormous contributions to reducing the state's road toll. In its focus specifically on the post-crash response – the system of care that kicks in once a person is injured – *From Roadside to Recovery* in no way diminishes the importance of these other components. Our seemingly selective attention to early injury prevention activities and trauma-related policies comes because these proved inseparable from the evolution of the VSTS – they involved similar organisations and people, used similar methods, and one was contingent on the other. But as we have tried to portray throughout this book, injury control requires complex adaptive systems with many integral components all working in concert.

We pay tribute, and offer our thanks to the many people and organisations who have contributed to the VSTS and to telling this story. There seems much to learn from it. We also hope it will guide and inspire – showing what is possible when a community is determined to address the tragedy, and cost, of road trauma. It is literally life changing.

Peter Bragge & Russell Gruen

July 2018

Chapter 1

AWAKENING

It is inevitable in this complex world
that individuals must abide by legislation
which is enacted in the interests
of society as a whole.

*(Brian Dixon, Liberal Member of Parliament and
Chair of the Road Safety Committee 1969–1970,
Dec 2 1970)*[1]

In 1905, Thomas Hall became the first recorded road fatality in Victoria after he was knocked down by the millionaire confectioner Macpherson Robertson. By the 1920s road fatalities were commonplace, and between 1945 and 1970 road deaths rose alarmingly and tragically as the number of cars on the road increased.[2]

Between 1960 and 1970 the number of road deaths in Australia was only 388 less than the total number of Australians killed during World War II. And as in war, more than half of those killed on the roads were young people in their prime, less than 30 years of age. Furthermore, per-capita road fatality rates were twice those of Great Britain, and higher than in the United States,[3] making many wonder what was different that made Australia's roads particularly hazardous.

The Victorian Government and the medical profession recognised they had a serious problem. By 1969, when Victoria's road deaths exceeded 1000 for the first time, a Victorian Parliamentary Road Safety Committee had been established (Appendix 1 lists all Inquiries conducted by the Committee),[4] the Australian Medical Association had released a road safety policy,[3] and the Royal Australasian College of Surgeons (RACS) had formed its Road Trauma Committee, which would become a pivotal contributor to road trauma prevention initiatives from the 1970s onwards.[3,5,6]

In 1970, Victorians were also exposed to a seminal newspaper campaign that "created a public climate of concern and became a press landmark in social responsibility"[3] by forcing the issue of road trauma graphically onto the public agenda. For almost 50 years to the present day, highly visible road safety messages would dominate roadside signage, major sporting events and print media, radio and television.

Road deaths would drop by almost 75 per cent. A methodical, relentless, research-driven campaign stopped thousands of lives from being destroyed.

Victorians today need little convincing that road trauma is a major public policy concern, and that a range of actions must be taken. In fact, the latest road safety strategy of the Victorian Transport Accident Commission is entitled 'Towards Zero,' signalling that the once unimaginable target of zero road deaths is a sufficiently realistic goal to motivate the population.[7]

On the back of successful world-first road safety legislation, government officials now know they can enact, without political obfuscation, legislation that makes a difference. It was the combination of an aware public, a motivated and equipped medical profession, and empowered policy-makers, that paved the way for a whole new trauma response system in Victoria – and the creation of a model that is being adopted around the world.

This chapter tells the story of the public campaigns and the legislative changes for which Victoria became a global leader, focusing on three critical road safety issues: seat belts, alcohol and speed.

"Declare war on 1034"

Victoria's number of road deaths for 1969 became the clarion call for a campaign by *The Sun News Pictorial*, later applauded as "the most successful newspaper campaign of the 20th century."[8] Spearheaded by the editor of *The Sun*, Harry Gordon, the newspaper launched the campaign on November 13, 1970 with a blistering editorial:

> **Declare War on 1034: Let's end this grim harvest of tragedy**
>
> In the seven weeks between now and the end of 1970, 160 people are expected to die on Victorian roads. Most of these victims, the victims for whom there will be no New Year, are probably reading this newspaper this morning. A chilling thought, yes. But we'll adjust to it. We always do. We, as a community, have developed a strange and unattractive talent: we accept as normal a rate of road slaughter that is the worst in the world. On Monday mornings, after each weekend's lunatic harvest of lives is counted, the same sincere adjectives – "appalling, shameful, irresponsible" – are paraded by the same sincere people. Then we think about other things, most of us, until the same sorry ritual occurs a week later. And all the time we are steadily, losing our capacity to be shocked, to be angry . . . The Sun's Ten Thirty Four campaign is an attempt to jolt people, to set a personal challenge for every driver. Ten Thirty Four isn't just the road toll figure for 1969.

It is a symbol of the dreadful carnage that makes this State, statistically, the most dangerous place on earth for drivers . . . Drivers can do it, if they concentrate on living through every day, every journey . . . We can all do it, if we work hard at staying alive. After all, we don't have to behave like lemmings, intent on steady self-destruction. Or do we?[9]

The campaign ran daily from November 13, 1970 until the end of the year. Graphic images and accompanying articles built upon the emotive theme of the editorial with in-depth descriptions of road trauma and passionate pleas regarding road safety.

The campaign used multiple strategies to impact readers, including a column by an author using the pseudonym 'Death,' stories of catastrophic injury, and stories of survival from use of seat belts. Death was having the time of his life:

Where the Young Die Good

You, in your world, would say the good die young. I say the young die good . . . They die good – in an inferno of speed and skid and scream . . . Bore me a bit, these young people. Always looking for me. Still, they help me top the 1034. I need only nine people a week. I'll be back in this column. So stay with me. I may need you, or you, or . . .[10]

The campaign brought to life those who were losing their lives:

The Princess Who'll Sleep Forever

NURSES at PANCH – the Preston and Northcote Community Hospital – call Sandra Russell "the Sleeping Princess". But Sandra, 23, isn't a "princess". She's a typist-receptionist from Donnelly Court, Pascoe Vale, the eldest of a family of six children, a part-time ballet student and a ballroom dancer who has won two medallions. And she's not "sleeping". She's a road accident victim who will never recover. Two years ago – on the night of November 23, 1968 – Sandra was thrown into the windscreen of a car driven by one of her brothers. She wasn't wearing a seat-belt. Her face was "cut to pieces" and her skull, pelvis and collarbone were broken . . . Sandra's brain is damaged beyond repair and although her eyes are open, she will never really "see" or be fully conscious again. She can suck elementary foods through a tube – and that's all. She can't move, can't communicate or – according to her doctors – recognise anyone or anything. But her condition can only, eventually, deteriorate – it can never improve. "I have come to accept that now", Sandra's mother, Mrs Beryl Whelan, said yesterday . . . "But you keep hoping and praying for a miracle. I was sure Sandra said 'Mum' to me once – but the doctors said I must have imagined it . . . It's not only the people who get killed", she said, close to tears. "It's the young people whose lives are ruined – the beautiful young people who are crippled and scarred. And their families, their brothers and sisters, their mothers and fathers who can never be the same again . . ."[11]

The campaign also used a town, Sea Lake, to illustrate graphically just what the toll represented. Sea Lake had a population of 1050. The newspaper asked its readers to imagine a disaster that painfully and bloodily killed all but 16 of the town's population. A shocked and outraged public would be screaming for an explanation, for a reason. The shocking truth was that the disaster was real; just not instantaneous or concentrated in one town. Nonetheless Sea Lake high school teacher Mike Nihill told his pupils that one of them would die every six years if the road toll didn't come down. The students were asked to imagine the town; their parents, their friends, all dead. This,

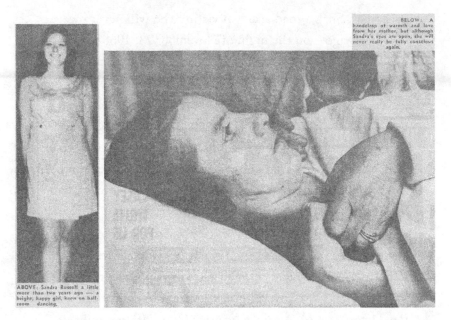

Sandra Russell, "the princess who'll sleep forever", before and after her accident
The Sun, November 26 1970, p.3

wrote the newspaper, was what had happened on Victorian roads the previous year. Road victims were not just a list of names, but the kind of cross-section which made up a small country town. "We destroy a town like Sea Lake every year. Make some sense out of that, if you can," it wrote.[13]

The newspaper was relentless. On Saturday, 28 November 1970, it predicted, challengingly:

> **Some of Us Won't Live**
>
> IT WILL be a beautiful weekend . . . warm and sunny. Just the weekend to spend some time on the beach, to work on the garden, to take a picnic in the park. The most depressing feature about this weekend is that a number of us won't survive. Some people who are reading this probably will die on the roads before Monday morning. Last year during these last

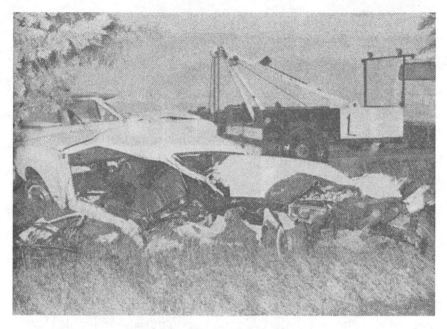

"Saved By Her Seat-Belt".
The caption accompanying this image reads: "Annie Sorbie, 56, was in the Royal
Melbourne Hospital last night. She is lucky . . . she could be dead. But thanks
to common-sense and a seatbelt, she escaped from the car smash
early yesterday with internal injuries . . . Ambulance men who pulled
her from the wreck said she owed her life to her seatbelt."[12]
The Sun, December 29 1970, p. 17

five weeks before December 31 there was a vintage harvest of
death on Victoria's roads. In that time 120 people died in car
accidents. All of them thought "It can't be me."[14]

It was a prophetic article. After 11 people were killed in a single
weekend, a senior policeman and a psychologist were asked to try
and explain. Both put responsibility squarely with driver attitudes.
Acting Chief Police Commissioner Mr Reg Jackson railed against
the "idiocy" and the "foolish exhibitionism" of many drivers. The
psychologist agreed, attributing what he called "highway homicide"

to intolerance, anger, aggression, fear, depression and uncontrolled frustration. He said that exhibitionism – taken to the point of stupidity – stemmed from these factors.[15]

The newspaper explained how the police catalogued road deaths: "Police action nil. Driver deceased." It explained that this bald notation referred to accidents in which drivers killed themselves by hitting trees or posts, losing control on bends or turning over – or colliding with another vehicle, killing themselves and someone else:

> Whatever the cause, any action open to police was cancelled
> because the people involved were DEAD.[16]

As the close of 1970 neared, the newspaper quoted the road manager of the National Safety Council of Victoria, Mr Frank Harris, tipping who victim number 1034 would be. "Mr 1034 will probably die on his way home from an office party this week," he said, alluding to the odds being weighted very much towards the attitude of male drivers.[17] He was close. At around 7 pm on December 16 1970, a male youth approximately 18 years old became the 1034th person to die on Victoria's roads that year when his bicycle collided with a car.[18]

The Sun also quoted the leader of the Victorian Country Party, Mr Ross-Edwards, as saying that one migrant ship was required for Victoria each year merely to replace the number of people killed on the roads: "We are slaughtering each other virtually every day," he said.[19] As the 1970 summer holiday period neared, and its prophetic toll of horror, the newspaper ratcheted up its desperate attempt to break through the inexplicable inability of people to think rationally when driving a car. The "it won't happen to me" barrier seemed impenetrable:

When Death is a Second Away

YOU have a second to live. You are going to die in a painful, agonising way, and you know it. No matter what you do, it's too late. You're dead. This story to an extent is a work of fiction. It has to be, because you can't interview a corpse . . . but you can establish some facts: It took about one second to kill most of them. If they were motorists, their bones did not just break, but shattered as their car – like the cars on these pages – underwent the almost unbelievable transformation from gleaming paint-work and chrome to splintered and torn metal. Whatever they collided with, the engine block, the heaviest part of the car, crashed back on to them, crushing them like a raw egg in a vice. And, of course, they didn't mean to die. There are very few suicides in cars. They died with that last terrible flash of amazement and terror.[20]

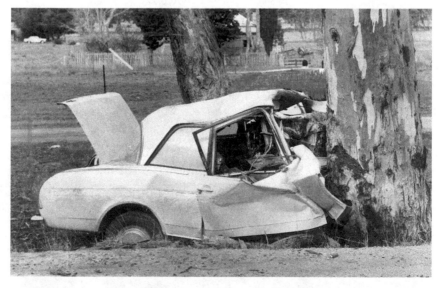

"Three young footballers died when this car ran off a country road and hit a tree"
The Sun, December 18 1970, p. 27

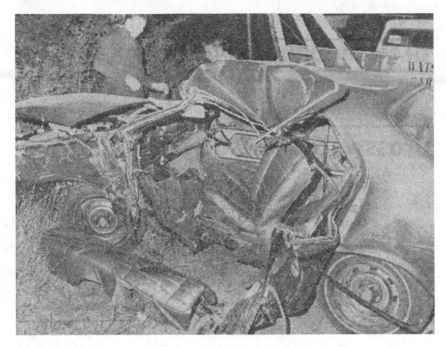

"A young couple died when this car smashed into
a power pole at Lower Plenty in February."
The Sun, December 18 1970, p. 27

Other features of the campaign included:

- daily road toll updates comparing 1970 with the previous year;
- road safety tips, quizzes and warnings, including broadcast warnings after horse racing meetings;[21]
- publication of readers' letters advancing suggestions for cutting the road toll;
- promotional posters distributed to 3500 members of the Victorian Automobile Chamber of Commerce, service stations, schools, shire councils, betting shops, public bars, and factories;[21,22]
- medallions and cash awards given to drivers showing courtesy on the road and cash prizes for readers whose letters were published;[9] and

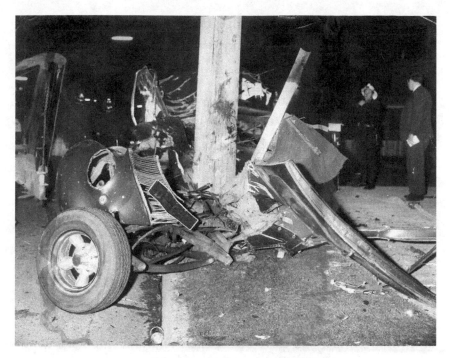

"Four youths died when this hot rod crashed into
a power pole at Box Hill in August."
The Sun, December 18 1970, p. 27

- accounts of observed examples of bad driving,[23] including
not wearing seat belts.[24]

It became a very emotive time in the media.[25] *The Sun* was the
widest circulating newspaper in Victoria, reaching over 645,000
people every day.[26] It set the pace for other sections of the media to
follow both in Victoria and interstate, as described by Professor Frank
McDermott, Surgeon and Chair of the Road Trauma Committee
from 1982–1996:

> Members of the media worked in a concerted attack. Day
> after day press, radio, and television campaigns were sustained
> in Melbourne, Sydney, and Adelaide. At a lighter level, a

commercial television network agreed to the Road Trauma Committee's suggestion that the police heroes of television drama wear seat belts.[3]

There were many examples. A 1970 feature article by *The Age* pressed the Government to accept the *Road Trauma Committee's* recommendations for the compulsory wearing of seatbelts; Donald Gibb and Donald Hossack from the *Road Trauma Committee* instigated the Victorian 'Belt up and Live' campaign in mid-1970, which used newspaper editorials, television and talkback radio to highlight the terrible consequences of road traffic injuries;[27] and the National Safety Council started a 'safety belt club' on September 10, 1970, which could be joined by anyone who had survived or avoided injury in an accident by using a seat belt. Members displayed red and white bumper and glove box stickers to promote the 'Buckle up your seat belt and live' campaign message;[28] and the Commonwealth Department of Shipping and Transport, in conjunction with the Road Safety Councils of Australia, produced a national 1970 television advertisement 'Please Wear Your Seat Belt,' featuring vision of dangerous driving, followed by police loading a dead body from an accident scene into a van.[a][29]

Given a strong and positive lead, the community showed it was willing to mobilise itself for war on the road toll. Individuals, radio and television stations, local councils, churches, schools, sporting clubs and private companies all engaged with this cause. Of all the arresting images in the 1034 campaign, the most emblematic was that of 1000 schoolchildren lying down in the main street of Red

---

[a] http://www.youtube.com/watch?v=Tc7_z4CH-iM

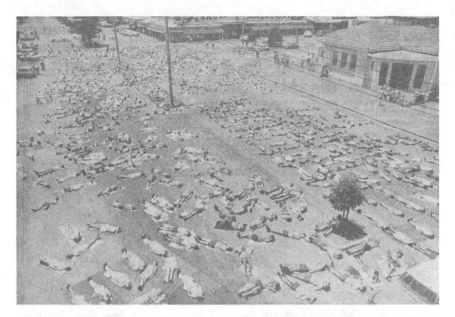

Iconic image from "The War on 1034" campaign; there were not enough children
to represent the 1034 people who had died on Victorian roads
The Sun, November 24 1970, *front page*

Cliffs, near Mildura, to represent the 1969 road toll. The organisers
had wanted 1034 to lie down, but ran out of children at 975.[30,31]

Buckling up

Declare War on 1034 had its genesis three years earlier, in 1967, when
the Victorian Parliamentary Road Safety Committee was established.[4]
In 1969, the Committee released its third report, 'Investigation into
the desirability of the compulsory fitting and the compulsory wearing of seat belts', which included a key recommendation:

> The Committee is convinced that no matter how much the
> public is exposed to education in the use of seat belts, apathy,
> lack of interest and lack of concern will mean that many people

will not wear them. The Committee therefore recommends
that all occupants of motor vehicles should be required to wear
seat belts within a maximum period of two years.[32]

There was already evidence available on the clear, positive, impact of compulsory wearing of seatbelts. Since 1967 they had been mandatory for all vehicles involved in the construction of the Snowy Mountains Hydro-Electric Scheme, which had previously recorded many deaths on the perilous mountain access roads and tracks. The road toll on the Scheme began falling as soon as the wearing of seatbelts was made compulsory, with failure to comply cause for instant dismissal. The Scheme's commissioner, Sir William Hudson, made the ruling after seatbelts saved the lives of two engineers during a work visit to Norway, where seatbelts had become standard (though not yet mandatory) fittings in cars.

However, despite the Committee being formed upon a foundation of political bipartisanship on road safety,[4] and strong evidence from the US, Europe and the Snowy Scheme in Australia showing that the wearing of seatbelts would reduce road trauma casualties,[33] the recommendation was initially met with political opposition, the main objection being that compulsory seatbelts infringed individual liberty.[34] It seemed the recommendation was also up against the belief that "many motorists did not feel sufficiently vulnerable to death or injury under normal driving conditions."[33]

The obstinacy wasn't helped by the most senior Victorian Government politicians of the day – the Premier, Sir Henry Bolte, and his Deputy, Sir Arthur Rylah – initially siding with civil libertarians who objected to the 'compulsory' element of the seatbelts proposal.[25,27] According to Peter Batchelor, Labor Minister for Transport from 1999–2006:

... the cabinet had already decided on the matter and they had
no intention of making seatbelt wearing compulsory ... neither
the Government nor the Opposition was likely to become
a public advocate of this course, despite the fact that the
committee, which included representatives from all parties, had
been unanimous in its recommendations. (August 7 2007)[25]

The recommendation fell on barren soil. After nine months
there was no action, no response from the Government.[3]

However, such opposition was met with sustained pressure from
other politicians and the medical profession, who were intent on
realising mandatory seat belt legislation. Walter Jona, who chaired
the Parliamentary Road Safety Committee from 1967–1973, led the
charge politically. He was a member of the ruling Liberal (conservative) Party at the time, but worked to promote the mandatory seat belt
laws with Committee members of all political persuasions including
Frank Wilkes, Deputy Leader of the opposition Labor Party, and Sir
Percy Byrnes, the Leader of the Country Party, as well as his Liberal
Party colleagues Brian Dixon, Murray Hamilton and Bill Fry:

Committee members from both sides of politics undertook
a campaign to win public support for this concept, and to
roll the political orthodoxy of the time. Walter Jona and his
committee colleagues approached the media in 1970. (Peter
Batchelor, August 7 2007)[25]

The Road Trauma Committee of the Royal Australasian College of
Surgeons, then led by Sir Edward (ESR) Hughes as Chairman and
Grayton Brown as Deputy Chairman,[5] joined the cause:

... the Road Trauma Committee began its efforts to counter
Parliamentary inertia, to make the community aware of the

life-saving value of seat belts, and to persuade the Government
to introduce legislation for compulsory wearing.[3]

Other supporters of the legislation included the Australian Medical
Association, the Victorian Police Surgeon, the Royal Automobile
Club of Victoria and the National Safety Council.[35] These lobbying
efforts fueled *Declare War on 1034*:

Awareness 'can change laws'

Community awareness could play a great part in cutting the
road toll, Mr Brian Dixon, MLA, told a road safety seminar
last night . . . Commenting on *The Sun*'s War on Ten Thirty
Four campaign, Mr Dixon said: "I believe it will have a
tremendous influence on road legislation. It could influence the
Government to act on reports by bodies like the Road Safety
Committee instead of putting them to one side." He said the
Government had a "very onerous" responsibility to make the
wearing of seat belts compulsory . . . Mr Dixon said the Liberal
Party was still considering whether to make the wearing of seat
belts compulsory, but he "prayed to God" that they did.[36]

Doctor: Why in hell won't they do it?

People who drink and drive get hurt and killed. People who
refuse to wear belts get hurt and killed. And they are the two
major factors. "So you make people stop drinking and driving,
you make them wear belts, and at least half the road toll is
solved . . . Why the hell won't they do it." (November 16 1970)[37]

Church leaders also joined into the debate, with Rev. Gordon Powell
of Scot's Church arguing that most responsible Victorians welcomed
Government action to curb the road toll:

The selfish minority must be ignored when they scream
about human rights and civil liberties, but . . . don't seem to

care about the hundreds of lives which will be lost if such legislation is not passed and enforced. (November 30 1970)[38]

The executive vice-president of the Victorian Automobile Chamber of Commerce, Mr A. M. Kelly, warned in *The Sun* that Victoria was in danger of losing on the roads the equivalent of a battalion in Vietnam:

> The tragedy is that the battleground is on our own doorstep, and as citizens we have not done nearly enough to save people from themselves. (December 16 1970)[39]

The campaign had grown from the lone voice of a newspaper editor to a chorus of recognised community leaders. And it worked.

On 2 December 1970, the Legislative Assembly passed legislation making it compulsory for Victorians to use safety belts in cars in which they were fitted. The law was to take effect from 1 January and the penalty for not wearing a seat belt was to be a $20 fine. The Bill also made it compulsory for new and second-hand cars to be fitted with seat belts before they were sold.[40] During Parliamentary debate, Sir William Fry of the Liberal party, who served on the Road Safety Committee from 1967–1976, praised *The Sun* for *"the splendid publicity campaign it has waged in support of this measure"*, noting also that the campaign had already led to an increase in drivers wearing seatbelts.[1] Brian Dixon, Liberal Member of Parliament and Chair of the Road Safety Committee between 1969–1970, used the same debate to directly address the civil libertarian argument against the legislation, emphasising it as an important precedent:

> It could well be said that this Bill is the forerunner of other measures which will be introduced where the interests of society are considered to be more important than the views of an individual. (December 2 1970)[1]

On 19 December 1970, in a letter to *The Sun*, Dixon reminded readers that wearing a seatbelt reduced the likelihood of injury by 50 to 80 per cent, depending on impact and speed.[41]

The Motor Cars (Safety) Act 1970 passed through the Upper House on 22 December.[42] On New Year's Day, 1971, Victoria became the first jurisdiction in the world to make wearing seat belts compulsory.[3]

The Sun editorialised:

> . . . Politicians say that one important effect of the 1034
> campaign has been the creation of a climate of concern,
> which has enabled them to propose sterner road laws on the
> wearing of seat belts and on drunken driving . . . The College
> of Surgeons Road Trauma Committee has written to us
> about it. So have numerous politicians. School teachers have
> set projects which were imaginative variations on the 1034
> theme. From it all has emerged the message that, despite the
> intense slaughter that has occurred on our roads, we are not
> a community of insensitive road zombies, we DO care very
> deeply, and just about all of us realise that we CAN make a
> personal contribution to road safety . . . If we leave a little
> earlier, drive a little slower, wear seat belts, refuse to drive
> after we've been drinking, if we all keep THINKING about
> surviving, we can do it. On this first day of the New Year, we
> should make it our resolution – and our personal challenge.
> (January 1 1971)[43]

In addition to the intense lobbying and media pressure, this legislation was also facilitated by the structure of the Australian political system; a federation of states. It meant a single state, like Victoria, could drive its own agenda and not be hamstrung by the far more onerous – and perhaps at the time, impossible – task of nationwide change.[44]

Even so, viewed in its political context, *Declare War on 1034* was cleverly harnessed by politicians to connect the largest and most important group of road safety stakeholders – the public – to previously hidden sectors of the community that had been dedicated to improving road safety for many years. The public was the audience rather than the initial target. *Declare War on 1034* was aimed at shaping public opinion enough to embolden the Victorian State Government to pursue a legislative endpoint. The passage of the mandatory seat belt law showed that this was a successful strategy. Walter Jona's words in parliament epitomise how the 1034 campaign connected Government and community:

> The Government and the community have a joint
> responsibility to control both the number of deaths and the
> number of casualty accidents. (December 2 1970)[1]

Declare War on 1034 was immediately successful in reducing the road toll. In November 1970, there were 67 road deaths, compared to 94 the previous November. This was enough to bring down the national Australian road toll – even though November road deaths in New South Wales, Queensland, Tasmania, South Australia, the Northern Territory and the Australian Capital Territory were higher than the previous year.[45]

The Victorian Road toll for 1970 was 1077: 56 less than the total projected by road safety statisticians. On New Year's Day, 1971, *The Sun* wrote on its front page:

> FIFTY-SIX people are walking around Victoria with a second
> chance. They might not have been alive for the first day of the
> New Year. Their lives were saved during the 1034 campaign,
> which dramatically changed Victoria's road-toll pattern in

the last seven weeks of 1970. Supt. H L Hookey, in a letter published in The Sun today, points out that another 700 people who would normally have been maimed or hurt during those seven weeks, are today unscathed. But maybe that was not the campaign's major achievement. Its great success was that it convinced people that they don't have to accept without question a rising road toll. They became involved. They cared. They did something. Responsibility and courtesy made a comeback. (January 1 1971)[43]

The newspaper continued its appraisal on page 8:

... any serious student of the road toll MUST consider the results of one of the most sustained publicity campaigns – and, we think, one of the most significant – in recent history. The message of the campaign has been simply this: If every one of us concentrates on staying alive, Victoria CAN cut the road toll drastically. Australia has had the worst road-death record per head of population in the world. And Victoria has had the worst record of any State in Australia. But we know now, after just seven weeks, that we can become a comparatively safe place. The Victorian president of the National Safety Council suggests that, on the evidence of 1034, we could become one of the safest States in the world. (January 1 1971)[43]

Surveys showed that, following the introduction of the legislation and associated enforcement measures, the rate of seat belt wearing in Victoria rose from 25% to 75% by May 1971. Reductions in deaths, the severity of head, spinal, pelvic, chest, abdominal and other injuries from road traffic accidents, and the probability of being thrown from the vehicle in a road traffic accident, were reported in the ensuing years.[3,33,46] Notably, in 1979, through analysis of road accident fatalities and injury data from 1955–1977, Frank McDermott and

Douglas Hough showed that the 1970 compulsory seat belt legislation led to a significant reduction in driver and passenger fatality rates that was sustained for all 7 post-legislation years.[47]

Mandatory seat belt legislation was subsequently introduced in New South Wales in October 1971, and all other Australian states by January 1972.[3] Data from other Australian states following the introduction of mandatory seat belt laws were similar to Victoria's, demonstrating 15–20% reduction in occupant fatalities:

> The number of traffic accident fatalities in Australia was contained below the record level of 3798 in 1970, in each of the seven succeeding years, despite increases of over 1.5 million in population and 2 million in motor vehicles . . . Over the years 1971 to 1977, some 4200 more people would have been killed had the trend from 1960 to 1970 continued.[33]

Many factors contributed to the success of seat belt legislation, including the installation of suitable belts in cars, favourable community attitudes, willingness of legislators to act in the face of expected public opposition, and ease of enforcement.[3,33]

The success of the Victorian seat belt legislation had international as well as national impact, with similar legislation being adopted in many other countries,[33] and Victoria was noted in a United States report on the effectiveness of seat belt laws.[35] Even now, with air bags commonplace, the importance of the seat belt remains; air bags and seat belts both reduce the occupants' impact against objects within the car, but only the seat belt prevents ejection from the vehicle.

Subsequent legislative efforts focused on child restraints, as data showed that, unlike adults, deaths and injury patterns had not changed among children under 8 years of age, who were exempt from the initial seatbelt laws.[47,48] In 1976 Victoria became the first Australian state to introduce compulsory front seat child restraints. In 1981 it was recommended that the legislation be extended to rear seat child restraints. Child restraints in both front and rear seats are today compulsory nationwide, and child restraint designs used in Australia have been proven to provide "exceptional protection to child occupants in severe crashes."[4]

After his death on July 22, 2007, Walter Jona was remembered for his pivotal role in the passage of the world's first mandatory seat belt laws:

> . . . car seatbelts became mandatory in Victoria under his guidance and leadership, and that has been a far-reaching initiative which has saved, literally, the lives of tens of thousands of Australians. (John Brumby, Premier of Victoria, August 7 2007)[25]

> When Victorians, and indeed people around the world, click on their belts every day, they are clicking on a little bit of Walter Jona. (Ted Baillieu, Leader of the Opposition, August 7 2007)[25]

> My first knowledge of Walter Jona perhaps was not quite as pleasant as those of other members . . . As we were driving back from Wilsons Prom I was pulled over by a policeman. I did not have my seatbelt on. I tried of course to talk my way out of it. He said, 'Don't blame me, blame the politicians'. I was getting quite passionate, and I said, 'Who do I write to?', and he said, 'Walter Jona'. That was my first knowledge of Walter Jona, but I agree it was a very wise law. (Christine Fyffe, Liberal Member of Parliament, August 7 2007)[25]

I also recall back in those earlier days being involved in a very serious accident on the way to a game of football at Gellibrand River . . . I have no doubt that had it not been for the introduction of compulsory seatbelts I would have been seriously injured in that crash and possibly have lost my life. On the Road Safety Committee we often talk about the silver bullet we are always looking for in relation to the next wave of road safety reform in the State of Victoria . . . I say to Walter's family that a silver bullet was fired by Walter back in the 1970s when he introduced legislation into Parliament for the compulsory wearing of seatbelts in Victoria. There is no doubt that there are thousands of families out there today who are not heartbroken, who have not been broken up, who have never experienced trauma and who have never suffered a loss of life because of the initiative and the absolute intestinal fortitude he showed at the time in taking that legislation forward. (Terry Mulder, Liberal Member of Parliament and member of the Road Safety Committee, August 7 2007)[25]

Drink driving

Between 1965 and 1975, alcohol consumption per adult head of population in Australia increased by over 40%. Curbing the problem of alcohol abuse was challenging because of the culture of the time. It encroached on a particular national sensitivity: the social acceptance of both alcohol and binge drinking was deeply entrenched.[3]

For health professionals, the association between alcohol consumption and road accidents was both obvious and alarming. In 1957 pathologist Dr John Birrell was appointed as a police surgeon with special responsibility for investigating road accidents. Birrell had noted a clear increase in the numbers of serious accidents in the

Harry Gordon: The editor's conscience

By Melissa Merino

Two car crashes killing multiple teen-agers on successive weekends in 1970 was appalling enough for journalist Harry Gordon. But what upset him more was the public's blasé accep-tance.

"The Monday morning there was the horror story (but) by about Wednesday other things were beating along and no one was angry about it – and I felt particularly angry," he said.

For Harry Gordon, these fatalities – and the apathetic response – were a tipping point; two crashes too many the year after 1034 people had died on Victoria's roads.

Through an interview recorded with his long-time friend Bill Shannon, Harry explained that his anger motivated him to act. And in his position, as editor of The Sun News Pictorial, his actions reached a lot of people.

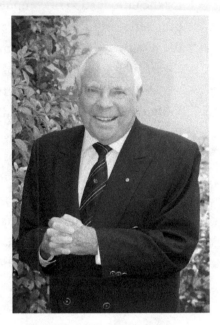

Harry Gordon, November 2006
Image supplied by Michael Gordon,
taken by Richard Webb

His 'Declare War on 1034' campaign started, he said, mainly to make people as angry as he was. "Most emphatically it was an intent to change behaviour on the road and change reactions to behaviour on the road," he said.

It ended up doing exactly that – playing a major role in Victoria being the first jurisdiction in the world to introduce compulsory seatbelts and seeing a significant drop in the road toll.

"We didn't set out to do it but . . . about half way through we realised the challenge was to make people accept regulations which otherwise and until then would have been unpalatable," he said.

Harry Gordon passed away in 2015 but the legacy of his war on 1034 lives on, in the changes it brought, the lives it saved and the lessons it held for 'behaviour change' campaigns that followed – particularly in how to condition a community to willingly accept change that it may initially resist.

"Mandatory seatbelts wouldn't have worked if Harry had not sensitised the community to embrace change," says Bill. "You can imagine the community reaction if the government had suddenly just thrust mandatory seatbelt legislation down its throat."

The 1034 campaign was so successful, it is why Bill – himself a behaviour change expert behind government Worksafe and water-saving campaigns among others – videoed Harry, creating a permanent record of his insights.

Particularly impressive, says Bill, is that Harry ran this classic 'behaviour change' campaign before the term was invented.

Rather than following any rulebook, Harry was writing the rules, simply by acting on his journalistic instincts, and his understanding of the Australian public and how to connect with them.

Even the rhyming catch-cry 'Declare War on 1034' reflects this, he says – catchy and memorable and designed to illicit an emotional response. "Nothing ever substitutes the importance of an emotional connection – and that takes an imagination like Harry's," Bill says. "You can throw money at a campaign and information at people but at the end of the day if you want change, you need to inspire people to change."

Harry himself said he came up with the concept 'Declare War on 1034' to appeal to the "schoolboy mentality" of readers, and the competitive instincts of people to "defeat" last year's toll.

This, says Bill, reflects a classic tenant of behaviour change campaigning used by agencies – including his own The Shannon Company – to shift people's actions: create an emotional connection by tapping into your audience's habits and beliefs.

"If you understand habits and beliefs you can have empathy and if you have empathy you can create an emotional connection, and if you create an emotional connection you can have action and normally if you have action you can have behaviour change," he says.

Appealing to his audiences' competitive nature is reflected in other creative facets of Harry's campaign, through awards for the best letters on road safety and prizes for young drivers who showed special initiative. He convinced the gatekeepers of Flemington racecourse and the MCG to run a 'Road Count' on scoreboards and with the cooperation of Melbourne's Lord Mayor had a giant barometer of the road toll erected in the city square.

Harry also worked with the community in other ways, taking the advice of a regional school principal to create what he remembers as the most novel aspect of the campaign – close to 1034 students and teachers laying down and being photographed from a cherry-picker to show people what that many bodies looked like.

Engaging people from the community demonstrated the connection he had made with the public, says Bill, but it also showed that Harry understood that for the campaign to be successful, he had to appeal to more than one audience.

Along with the readers of his newspaper, he was also targeting influencers and decision makers; his media colleagues and advertisers, police and ultimately the government. "I think they (politicians) saw it was being accepted and they were prepared to enact legislation", Harry said.

Bill says if politicians were worried they may lose votes by forcing people to wear seatbelts, by the time Harry had sensitised the community that was no longer a problem. "They were onside – they were all for it," he says.

Cooperation, said Harry, was one of the features of the campaign he most fondly remembered. The chemistry was right, he said, with support from the police, the Royal Australian College of Surgeons, many municipalities, sporting bodies and members of parliament.

"It was like a beautiful football team coming together for the last quarter," Harry said. "And we didn't even know for three quarters we were on the same side."

On reflection, Harry acknowledged there was no other campaign he could remember that had such "comforting" results or was so "resoundingly" successful. "But I don't feel smug . . . it's done nothing for my ego," he said. "I just think it was a damn good campaign."

hour after Melbourne's notorious 'six o'clock swill' and the high concentrations of alcohol in the blood of many victims. Birrell began what was probably the first public campaign to introduce compulsory random breath testing of motorists.[2]

Although a maximum legal blood alcohol concentration of 0.05% was established in 1966, it was several years before efforts to mitigate alcohol-associated trauma intensified. In November 1970, surgeon Donald Hossack, a member of the Road Trauma Committee and then consultant to the Melbourne City Coroner, released analysis showing that 86 of 171 driver fatalities had levels of alcohol between two and 10 times the legal limit. Breath tests were subsequently introduced by police in August 1971.[27] Further lobbying from the

**If you drink, then drive,
you're a bloody idiot.**
TAC

'Drink Drive Bloody Idiot' billboard from Victorian Transport
Accident Commission campaign
Image supplied by Clemenger Group with permission of the
Victorian Transport Accident Commission

RACS Road Trauma Committee followed, with mass media and public support. A page from *The Sun* newspaper, juxtaposing an article reporting calls for more alcohol breath tests with a beer advertisement, illustrates the cultural challenge faced in countering drink driving.[49]

Eventually, as for seat belts, legislation was enacted. On April 8, 1974, blood alcohol tests on all Victorian road crash casualties 15 years of age and over became compulsory.[50] Although the mandatory blood-taking law was repealed in 1991 (the legal onus is now on accident victims to allow a blood test),[4] compulsory blood alcohol-testing from 1974 to 1991 opened a critical window of data collection which was used to guide policymaking.

Frank McDermott and Peter Strang analysed blood alcohol test results from almost 43,000 road crash casualties and concluded in 1978 that alcohol was "the most important single contributing cause of serious road crashes and fatalities in Australia,"[3] with illegal blood alcohol concentrations found in 50% of driver fatalities, most frequently in males under 25 years of age.[50]

This led the RACS Road Trauma Committee to advocate for a further legislative countermeasure, as it had with mandatory seat

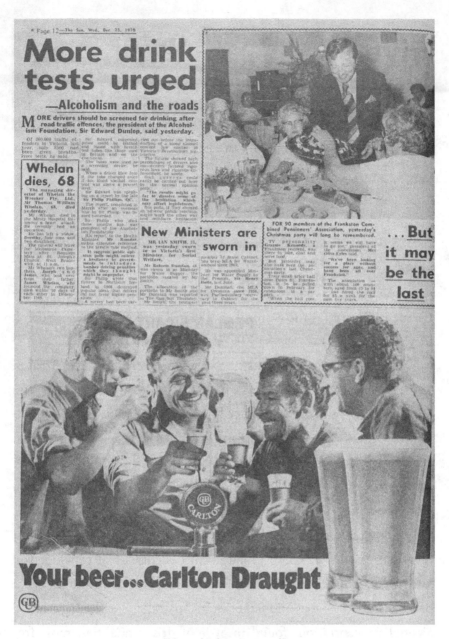

"More drink tests urged"
The Sun, December 23 1970, p. 12[49]

belt laws.[3] In July 1976, Victoria pioneered the implementation of Random Breath Testing (RBT) of motorists. This was noted in 1990 as a watershed in drink drive laws by criminologist Professor Ross Homel AO, because it was the first step in a sustained movement toward increased penalties and more rigorous enforcement in all parts of Australia.[51]

However, despite Victoria again pioneering road safety legislation, RBT enforcement efforts did not match those of other states. Homel described the introduction of RBT in July 1976 as a "daring initiative" given the beery culture of the time. But he said most of the daring seemed to have been spent on passing the law, with little left over for actual enforcement. Victoria's 19,006 breath tests conducted in 1977 paled in comparison to the nearly one million in the first year of RBT in New South Wales.[51]

Nevertheless, Victoria's RBT approach, which centred on intensified blitzes in areas of Melbourne, yielded promising results. The percentage of driver and rider fatalities who were over the legal blood-alcohol limit fell from almost 50% in the 1970s to 37% by 1982,[52] and accidents in blitz areas were reduced by more than 20%.[51]

After further substantial media support and political lobbying, legislation passed in May 1984 mandated zero blood alcohol for first year drivers. By 1990 this had been extended to all three probationary driving years.[4] Similar legislation followed in other Australian states.

However, more was needed. By the late 1980s the reduction in road deaths of people with a blood alcohol level exceeding 0.05 had levelled out. At the same time, research into Australian RBT strategies had begun to unlock critical insights into how such interventions might exert their influence. A review published in 1988 by Homel and colleagues, "Random breath testing in Australia: a complex deterrent", found that the apparent effectiveness of RBT was due to its preventative capacities rather than the detection of offenders, for which it was originally designed.[53] The true objective of RBT, therefore, was to create a perception among drivers that if they drink then drive, their apprehension was inevitable. As summarised in 1995 by Inspector Michael Moloney from the Traffic Alcohol Section of Victorian Police: "Whether that threat is real or otherwise is not the point, the point is whether the public believes it to be."[54]

To be successful, RBT had to be highly visible, rigorously enforced, credible, sustained, and well publicised.[51,53,54] In 1989, after lobbying by Victoria Police, RBT was re-structured accordingly.

The Transport Accident Commission (TAC) was pivotal to this restructure. Established in 1987, TAC is a state-owned Victorian Government enterprise operating as a commercial insurer funded by premiums and investment income generated on reserves. The TAC's accident compensation scheme combines no-fault and common law benefits to ensure everyone is covered regardless of fault, as well as allowing those who could prove fault to pursue further compensation through the courts.[55] The history of how TAC grew out of previously unsustainable compensation schemes is described in detail in Chapter 2.

Apart from the effective and efficient management of Victoria's accident compensation scheme, another of the TAC's ongoing primary objectives has been to reduce the incidence and cost of transport accidents.[55] This mandate, combined with the TAC's standing as a legislated monopoly transport accident compensation provider, positioned Victoria uniquely with a major funding body having a vested interest in improving road accident outcomes. Consequently, the TAC supported enforcement, promotion, healthcare and research since its inception.

The TAC funded key components of the restructured RBT program. In 1990, the TAC purchased 13 'booze buses' – dedicated vehicles facilitating highly visible and efficient roadside RBT by Victoria Police. These booze buses were a visible 'flagship' of the Victorian RBT effort and their use was another world first. The Government also tasked the TAC with publicising the RBT campaign.[54,56] How the TAC did this was to become a blueprint for road injury prevention campaigns.

The centrepiece of the seminal RBT campaign was a series of graphic television advertisements, costing $23 million,[57] screened on television between 1989 and 1992, all featuring the now famous tagline 'If you drink, then drive, you're a bloody idiot.'[58] The advertisement 'Girlfriend', launched December 12 1989,[b] depicted a badly injured young woman arriving at hospital after a crash and the driver, her drunk boyfriend, being confronted at the hospital by the girl's angry parents.[59] This was followed on September 12 1990 by 'Booze Bus,'[c] featuring drivers caught through 'booze buses' reacting to penalties for driving with a blood alcohol content above 0.05;[60] and on November 29 1992 by 'Joey,'[d] where two brothers leave a party, one of whom insists on driving despite being drunk.[61] The car rolls off the road, seriously injuring the driver and killing his brother.[58,62]

The television advertisements comprised about 70% of the campaign, with the balance spent on radio, press, outdoor advertising (including mobile billboards), pay television and cinema.[57,62]

---

[b] http://www.youtube.com/watch?v=TfhR5w5uYWs
[c] http://www.youtube.com/watch?v=J5_n5sgcbEc
[d] http://www.youtube.com/watch?v=goDczc2KXtE

The renewed RBT strategy increased the number of breath tests from about half a million in 1989 to over 1.1 million by 1991.[56] The percentage of drivers and riders killed with a blood alcohol content above 0.05, which had well exceeded 30% in the early 1980s, fell to 21% in 1992.[52,54]

Research into the effectiveness of the publicity campaign reported a 14% reduction in night-time crashes resulting in serious casualties, a statistically significant association between the level of advertising and crash reduction, and substantial cost savings largely due to the averted medical expenses.[57,62,63]

Results of the dual publicity/enforcement campaign were consistent with similar campaigns in other countries, such as New Zealand.[57] In New Zealand it was also shown that without advertising, RBT enforcement had little impact on the number of positive breath tests – in other words, media campaign effectiveness is greatest when it is linked to RBT enforcement. The TAC produced a further 29 drink-driving television advertisements between September 1993 and September 2006, [58] and a similar approach was also used for other campaigns, such as those focusing on speeding.

Speed kills

The Victorian Parliamentary Road Safety Committee produced five reports on speed limits, speed detection and speeding penalties between 1969 and 1995.[4] Although speed cameras were trialed in Victoria in 1985,[64] the state's first concerted speed camera program began in April 1990. Consistent with the formula underpinning the success of the drink driving strategy, TAC funded both enforcement, through their purchase of 54 radar mobile speed cameras for Victoria Police, and an intensive media campaign.[56,65]

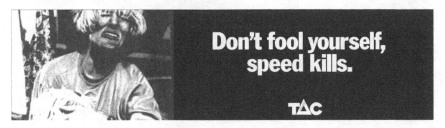

Speed kills billboard from Victorian Transport Accident Commission campaign
Image supplied by Clemenger with permission of the Victorian Transport Accident Commission

Three TAC advertisements were launched in 1990 on the theme "Don't Fool Yourself – Speed Kills."[62,66] 'Speed Cameras' (launched 4 April 1990)[e] was designed to counter the view that speed cameras are all about 'revenue raising'. A surgeon explains how speed cameras work, followed by vision of the surgeon in an operating theatre, to reinforce the consequences of speeding.[67] 'Beach road' (4 April 1990)[f] targeted drivers who justify their speeding by referring to the speed of other traffic. A mother mourns at a road accident scene where a speeding driver has hit and killed a young boy, as an ambulance officer explains that 'the faster you drive, the harder you hit and the more damage you do.'[68] 'Tracey' (12 September 1990)[g] focused on young, female provisional license drivers who tend to speed. A distraught young woman who was speeding mourns 'my best friend and I killed her' as her critically-injured friend leaves in an ambulance.[69]

Following the rollout of the speed cameras, their use increased from 250 hours in June 1990 to approximately 1500 hours or more per month in 1991. Consequently, the number of speeding offences

---

[e] http://www.youtube.com/watch?v=5hdekam-qNk
[f] http://www.youtube.com/watch?v=18jVzR86mCc
[g] http://www.youtube.com/watch?v=JnUOCNw7Urs

detected also rose dramatically, from 20,000 per month prior to July 1990 to up to 80,000 per month thereafter.[65]

Research undertaken by the Monash University Accident Research Centre (MUARC) concluded that the speed-limit campaign, in combination with other enforcement programs, including mandatory bicycle helmet wearing and lowering the freeway speed from 110km/h to 100km/h, resulted in a substantial reduction in Victorian road trauma.[63]

Fatalities dropped from 776 in 1989 to 396 in 1992. This was the largest reduction in Victorian history – the road toll had not been under 400 since 1948, when there were 87% fewer vehicles registered.[56]

Legislative and enforcement efforts against speed continued in Victoria throughout the 1990s and the turn of the century. In December 1996, Victoria Police deployed 60 new laser speed detectors.[56] A new 40km/h speed limit for school and shopping strip zones was also implemented in 2001–2002.[56] Speed limits and speed enforcement in Victoria are still regularly reviewed.[70,71]

Whereas any public opposition to seat belt and blood alcohol legislation had been based on infringement of civil liberties, the main objection to the use of speed cameras was that they were seen to be for revenue raising, rather than reducing road trauma. The revenue gathered through fines was perceived to be excessive and directed not to furthering road safety but instead to bolstering consolidated revenue.[64,72]

Other arguments mounted against speed cameras included the perception that speeding slightly in excess of the limit does not increase crash risk; that no opportunity is given to explain the circumstances of a speeding event; and that speed cameras are neither accurate nor reliable.[64]

In both 2006 and 2011 the Victorian Auditor General examined these concerns. It was concluded that road safety cameras were effective in reducing road trauma and their ongoing use was appropriate; revenue generation was not the primary purpose of the road safety camera program; the location of cameras was based on road safety objectives; and that while the accuracy of any system cannot be absolutely guaranteed, sufficiently reliable processes and controls were in place.[72,73]

Despite these findings, debate about the purpose and value of speed cameras has continued in Victoria. It is important to address these public concerns, as such negative perceptions have been seen to contribute to abolishment of photo radar programs, for example in British Columbia.[64] To this end, efforts to promote the evidence base and rationale behind speed camera enforcement are ongoing, for example through the Victorian Government 'Cameras Save Lives' website.[74]

The evolution of road safety advertising

The "drink drive bloody idiot" campaign of 1989 was the start of what would be a relationship over more than 20 years between the TAC, Sweeney Research, a market research company, and Grey Advertising, an advertising agency. Television advertising campaigns have been the staple, relentlessly drawing upon four principles: (1) Ensure that every ad leaves us thinking 'That could so easily be me'; (2) Be as shocking as you like; (3) Be as emotional as possible; and (4) Emphasise the link between drink/drive, speed, etc and real crashes.[75]

Realism and credibility of the message were key ingredients. The TAC has employed Australia's top film directors, often shooting commercials over three days with a hundred-strong cast, road closures and Police participation.[75] The large budgets needed reflected the Victorian Government's determination to tackle injury on the roads, and to use the TAC as the main vehicle for doing so. In the late 1980s the TAC was told to "stop this bloody carnage, this is crazy – you go and do it," according to Peter Hennessy from Sweeney Research.[76]

> If they made cheap and nasties it wouldn't haven't been anything like as effective. Because they wanted . . . real people that you and I can associate with . . . I can see him, or her, as a typical bike rider or pedestrian, or whatever, they're real people, and you get that real quality coming out that you can associate with. (Peter Hennessy, September 7 2015)[76]

Over the years, key personnel from Sweeney Research and Grey Advertising became deeply vested in the TAC advertising brand. And they took their custodianship of it very seriously. When the office of Jim Kennan, the Government Minister launching the TACs first advertising campaign, got wind of the TAC's first tagline – "if you drink then drive, you're a bloody idiot" – it was made clear that the Minister would not be saying the word 'bloody' and that the offending word should be removed. It was retained as the result of a convenient administrative error and the rest, as told by the brainchild of the slogan, Greg Harper, is history:

> I didn't want to be the first person to promote the word "bloody" on television . . . but the research favoured "bloody"; so . . . it went on to a thousand billboards and footy guernseys – and into marketing history.[77]

But the custodianship of the TAC advertising extended well beyond its launch. The TAC's 107 (and counting) TV commercials were the result of testing and re-testing of approximately 1000 advertising concepts. Peter Hennessy described "colossal" disputes between advertisers and market researchers as the passion for the brand spilled over, especially when attempts to 'refresh' the brand were made in the early 2000s. Such tinkering was fiercely resisted by Sweeney and Grey through their considerable influence on the upper echelons of the TAC:

> a lot of companies over time, if you look, they've destroyed their brand or given their brand hiccups when it was absolutely stupid. Some new marketing person comes in, 'oh yeah, I'm going to rejuvenate it, change the packaging' . . . Why? Oh, because we should . . . in most cases it doesn't work, consumers are creatures of habit. (Peter Hennessy, September 7 2015)[76]

The advertisers and market researchers recognised that this was not like, say, selling soap. It was a mission to convince large groups in society to rethink their perceived invincibility on the roads. Lives were at stake. Their investment in these campaigns was absolute:

> these people are bloody proud of TAC, they're proud of the achievements, don't you stuff up my TAC. That's my campaign, it's not someone else's campaign, I own it. (Peter Hennessy, September 7 2015)[76]

And Peter Hennessy recalled, each of their many victories was met with another target:

> I remember years ago . . . we'll set a target of 400, get it under 400. People were oh, yeah, bullshit, we'll never get that, but we'll aim for it. Then there's like 300, a big ask, you'll never get that. And of course now, I don't know how low you can go.[76]

The road toll was not the only indication of the campaign's impact. For example, the TAC produced several television advertisements in the 1990s on the theme 'Belt Up or Suffer the Pain.' Launched in March 1992, the first advertisement was 'Bones',[h] which targeted young people who believe it is 'un-cool' to wear seat belts.[62] A young woman not wearing a seat belt is thrown through the front window following an accident and later undergoes difficult physiotherapy.[78] Surveys conducted following this campaign indicated that people found it easier to encourage passengers to wear a seat belt, and over 80% of those surveyed insisted that everyone in the car wore a seat belt.[62]

This underlines the pivotal role of market research in the TAC's road safety campaigns. The TAC advertisements of the late 1980s and early 1990s were largely organic in their evolution, focusing on the simple delivery of a road safety message. From the mid 1990s, advertising content became progressively more sophisticated, in particular due to the influence of market research on the advertising development process, but also as a result of expansion of the scope of promotion activities. By 2006, Sweeney Research had conducted over 50,000 telephone surveys and over 1000 focus group or one-on-one interviews exploring Victorians' attitudes and behaviours regarding driving, including how they feel about road laws and their perception of the risks involved in breaking them.

Market research also became increasingly sophisticated. Advertising was developed in response to arguments against road safety enforcement initiatives that were identified in focus groups and interviews. The campaigns then became more extensive in scope, and employed different media and promotional strategies.

---

[h] http://www.youtube.com/watch?v=O8gUXBvffdk

The TAC's 2001 speed campaign epitomised this evolution. Market research found that drivers had difficulty accepting that reducing speed by 5km/h had a significant impact on road safety. Advertising concepts were developed to counter this view and publicise a sharp increase in police enforcement. The advertising concept was tested in focus groups. The resulting campaign aimed to dispel the myth that exceeding the speed limit by 5 to 10km/h is 'safe.' Based around the theme 'Wipe Off 5,' television, radio, print and billboard advertising was timed to coincide with Police enforcement; well recognised organisations such as the Collingwood Australian Rules Football Club were sponsored; and high-profile launches were held with senior politicians and the Police Minister to generate news publicity. These were accompanied by associated promotional activities such as distribution of posters and stickers at service stations, 'Wipe off 5' week, a major 'blockbuster' Australian Rules football match featuring half-time 'Wipe off 5' fireworks, and a media event involving star Australian Rules footballers. Following the campaign launch, telephone surveys evaluated the campaign's effectiveness. Fewer drivers admitted to speeding compared to a pre-campaign survey, more believed they would be caught speeding, fewer believed speed cameras were

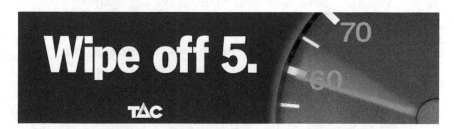

Wipe off 5 billboard from Victorian Transport Accident Commission campaign
Image supplied by Clemenger Group with permission of the Victorian
Transport Accident Commission

primarily a revenue raising tool, and the advertisement was positively received, especially among younger age groups.[79]

The return on TAC's substantial investment has driven growth in the TAC's media budget from $10 million in the 1990s to $22.5 million by 2012. Although a large amount is spent on television advertising, roughly 30% is spent on outdoor advertising (which has attracted criticism for potentially distracting motorists) and there is also considerable investment in sporting sponsorships.

In addition to seatbelts, alcohol and speed, TAC campaigns have covered driver distractions, drug driving, fatigue, motorcycle safety and the influence of parental role modelling on young driver behaviour. The campaigns have won major advertising awards, including at Cannes,[75] and have informed similar campaigns by other governments and in other languages, including those in China, the UK, South Africa and New Zealand.

Although a substantial part of the road safety landscape, TAC advertising has not been the only plank in the strategy to reduce road carnage in Victoria. In the early 2000s the State also invested in multifaceted road safety strategies based around the concept of a 'safe system,' recognising the need to address roads, people, vehicles and other factors in concert.[56] This led to the launch in November 2001 by the Victorian Government of 'Arrive Alive 2002–2007'.[70]

This package brought together increases in covert and flashless speed camera operations, a 50% increase in camera operating hours, introduction of a 50km/h general urban speed limit in January 2001, increased speed-related advertising, and restructure of speeding penalties.[72,80]

Analyses in 2004 estimated fatal crashes were reduced by 27%, equating to a saving of over 8 lives per month.[4,80] Similarly, 'Arrive

Alive 2008–2017' combined increased penalties for drink driving, a restriction to one peer passenger (aged 16–21) in the first year of probationary licenses, mandatory electronic stability control (ESC) in all new cars built after 31 December 2010, more targeted roadside drug testing stations and increased road funding.[56,70]

Recent road safety promotion strategies highlight further innovation and recognition of the emergence of new media. The TAC has run billboard advertisements in the background of video games on popular platforms such as Xbox 360™ and Playstation™.[75] In February 2011, a small Victorian town named 'Speed' was approached by the TAC with the idea of being renamed 'SpeedKills' for one month. The town's 40 residents agreed to promote the 'Rename Speed' campaign, designed to make speeding as socially unacceptable as drink driving. They participated in a television advertisement calling for 10,000 people to visit the Rename Speed Facebook Page, upon which the TAC would donate $10,000 to the local Lion's Club. The page subsequently attracted over 30,000 followers and TAC doubled its donation. A local farmer also changed his name to Phil 'Slow' Down for a month. The renaming attracted considerable media publicity.[81,82]

The TAC's campaigns have underscored the value of investing in powerful messages. Victorians can recall the specifics of slogans and key messages of TAC road safety advertisements 10 to 15 years after they have stopped airing – a recall that is well beyond the norm.[76]

This chapter has highlighted the synergistic roles of mass media campaigns and road safety legislation over five decades. The seat belt, alcohol and speed road safety campaigns highlight in a number of ways how community sentiment and, by extension, the views of legislators, can be influenced by mass media publicity. *Declare War on 1034* targeted legislators through public opinion, whereas '*Drink*

Snapshot: Other road safety strategies

Bicycle Helmets

In the late 1970s, bicycle helmet-wearing rates were less than 5%, whereas virtually all motorbike riders wore helmets, which became compulsory in 1961. Data from the Victorian Motor Accident Board from 1977–1979 showed that bicycle riders sustained more frequent and severe head injuries than motorcycle riders. The Victorian Road Trauma Committee of the Royal Australasian College of Surgeons, the Australian Medical Association and the Royal Automobile Club of Victoria spent the next decade agitating, with strong media support and coverage, for compulsory helmet-wearing legislation for cyclists.[83]

The legislation, another world first, was introduced into Parliament on 1 July, 1990.[4,83,84] Helmet wearing rates increased from 31% in March 1990 to 75% in March 1991, and insurance claims from bicyclists killed or admitted to hospital following head injury decreased by 48% and 70% in the first and second years. However, the large reduction in head injuries was not solely attributed to reduced risk of head injury in bicycle crashes – a reduction in the number of bicyclists involved in crashes, partly through a reduction in bicycle use, was also observed.[85]

As with other road safety legislative and enforcement measures, the issue of mandatory helmet wearing for cyclists has been controversial, and activist groups continue to campaign against these laws.[86] While they have tried to discredit the scientific evidence used to support helmet wearing, and argue against mandatory helmet use,[86–89] such arguments have been fiercely rebutted. Hagel and Pless (2006)[90] highlighted two independent systematic reviews, which concluded that bicycle helmets prevent head and brain injuries in a variety of crash situations.[90–92] There is also evidence and argument against the notion that cyclists wearing helmets take fewer (or greater) risks.[90,93]

Data from trauma registries does not support the claim that helmet use increases the risk of cervical spine injury.[89]

Drug Driving

1 December 2004 saw the passing of a new legislative framework in Victoria that prohibited driving under the influence of drugs and gave police the authority to conduct random drug tests (RDTs), using a 'drug bus' comparable to the 'booze bus.'[94] In a familiar sequence, Victoria was the first jurisdiction in the world to introduce the legislation. Other Australian States followed in the ensuing years,[95] and the strategy was underpinned by widespread TAC advertising.[96] In June 2014 the Victorian Government legislated to become one of the first jurisdictions in the world to define driving under the influence of drugs as an offence. This was in response to figures demonstrating that drivers with alcohol and drugs in their system are 23 times more likely to be killed in a crash than others, and that approximately 8 per cent of road deaths that involve alcohol also involve drugs.[97,98]

Vehicle Safety Features

The TAC took a novel approach to promoting car safety technologies. Instead of lobbying Government to legislate or developing regulations, they launched a campaign to mobilise the community to demand two important car safety features – electronic stability control (ESC), which uses computers to control braking when the driver loses control, thereby preventing 'fish-tailing,' and curtain airbags. Research by the Monash University Accident Research Centre showed these have a high-level benefit in reducing accidents and the severity of accidents.

The 'how safe is your car' website was launched in 2006 to promote the initiative.[99] At this time, less than 20% of Victorians had ESC in their cars. This rose to over 40% in 2008 and over 60% by 2011. Following the combined efforts of the TAC, Victoria Police, road and justice authorities, ESC was made mandatory in all new cars sold in Victoria – legislation that was subsequently adopted nationally.[100] A more recent focus has been on Auto Emergency Braking (AEB), which can alert the driver to an imminent crash and apply the brakes independently of the driver if the situation becomes critical.[99]

Drive Bloody Idiot' and *'Speed Kills'* combined enforcement with publicity to influence road users' behaviour. These campaigns spawned tailored road safety promotion strategies that continue to this day.

Teasing out the isolated and combined effects of publicity, legislation and enforcement on road safety outcomes is a complex task. Difficulties inherent in statistical modelling, and adjustment to account for concurrent activities has led to academic debate about what it is that makes road safety publicity campaigns effective.

One such debate is the effectiveness of emotional versus informational messaging. Critics of the TAC's advertising have argued that it should focus on modelling desirable behaviours rather than promoting fear.[57] Research on alcohol-related crashes found that campaigns emphasising legal deterrence may be more effective for eliciting individual behaviour change in the short term, whereas emotionally-intense campaigns emphasising personal and social costs may be more effective at garnering community support for introduction of legislation aimed at preventing injury.[57] Another review concluded that persuasive or emotive campaigns are more effective than informational-style campaigns, especially when they are underpinned by robust theoretical models and are combined with public relations and associated publicity.[101] This may explain both the investment by TAC in market research and its focus on emotive campaigns.

Notwithstanding the debate on specific advertising approaches, the examples presented in this chapter illustrate the TAC's considerable impact and reach. The very first TAC advertisement had immediate impact and sparked substantial media debate. The unchanged TAC logo has become a fixture on the roadside and in living rooms, and the TAC YouTube channel currently has over 16,000 subscribers and over 35 million views.[75,102]

Although the influence on legislation of '*Drink Drive Bloody Idiot*' and '*Speed Kills*' was not as obvious as it was in the case of *Declare War on 1034*, these campaigns are understood to have altered individual behaviour and contributed to shifting public opinion:

> . . . mass media can play an "agenda-setting" role by influencing public perceptions of the importance of social issues, such as alcohol-impaired driving (AID). As media coverage increases the perceived importance of the AID problem, public support for actions to address it may also increase . . . According to some authors, using the mass media to influence social policies offers much larger potential benefits than attempting to change individual behaviour.[57]

Key lessons can be drawn about the importance of mass media. In addition to its value in generating community awareness, publicity is synergystic with enforcement and legislation. This synergy can be enhanced through systematic, research-driven methods for developing road safety campaigns. The bi-directional nature of this interaction is illustrated by a study on the influence of media on drink driving behaviour and policy response, which concluded that while substantial direct media effects on legislation and behaviour were present, "the direct effect of media on behaviour was no longer significant when the effect of legislation on behaviour was controlled."[103] The authors of this study also found from related research that:

> considerable evidence that media attention to public problems influences the nature and magnitude of policy responses to these issues . . . in addition to their indirect influence on the policy agenda through the public agenda, the mass media were often found to influence policy makers directly, as policy makers often infer the public agenda from the media

agenda. This tendency makes policy makers particularly susceptible to media coverage of public problems for two main reasons . . . both the media and the public expect policy makers to focus on resolving public problems . . . media attention to public problems opens a window of opportunity for political gain.[103]

If mass media's influence on the community and its legislators was a catalyst for action on road safety, political bipartisanship was a key ingredient in the ensuing reaction. This was established from the creation of the Parliamentary Road Safety Committee in 1967:

> The bipartisan composition and support of the Committee enables legislative changes to be recommended that may otherwise be politically contentious for individual parties to initiate. These changes have inevitably played a significant role in the reduction of road related fatalities and injuries in Victoria. Overall the Committee has played a key role in Victoria's road safety history.[4]

According to Peter Batchelor, this Committee "set a trend that continues through to today where road safety measures must continue to be delivered in a bipartisan fashion" (August 7 2007)[25] Although seat belt and other laws were delayed by political debate and intransigence, this was as much within parties as between them.

The Victorian Parliamentary Road Safety Committee ceased to exist on April 21, 2015, when it merged with the Law Reform, Drugs and Crime Prevention Committee to become the Law Reform, Road and Community Safety Committee. That it became redundant is perhaps most telling of what the Road Safety Committee achieved in its 48 years. No Victorians would doubt the importance of injury as a public policy problem:

We have heard about Walter Jona's contribution in terms of the seatbelt legislation. It made a great difference. It was controversial at the time, but he showed great courage in pursuing that legislation. It also inspired a great tradition here in this state of Victoria, where we have gone from being one of the worst jurisdictions in the world per capita in terms of road-related deaths to being one of the best. We now have people from jurisdictions across the world coming to Victoria to see what we are doing. That compulsory seatbelt legislation created a tradition and was followed by random breath testing, the Transport Accident Commission ads changing the whole mindset of the community as far as road safety goes, and of course random roadside drug testing, which is now being emulated by other jurisdictions in Australia and across the world. Each of those measures was initially controversial, but Victoria has led the way. I think Walter Jona, through his work on the seatbelt legislation, inspired a tradition here in this state for which we stand out as a beacon to the rest of the world. (Andre Haermeyer, Labor Member of Parliament, August 7 2007)[25]

Chapter 2

MONEY

I often like to tell the story of the TAC being
the son of two hopelessly insolvent parents,
who actually did very well.

*(John Bolitho, former TAC Senior Legal Counsel,
December 16 2014)*[104]

Insurance – like tax – is perceived as a necessary evil of modern life. Most people only ever hear from insurance companies when a bill is due or to be informed that premiums are to rise. Insurance is paid begrudgingly, because unlike comparable expenses, return on investment is almost always intangible; its value is only realised at times of crisis that are fortunately rare or non-existent – house fires, car theft or the unexpected death of a loved one.

When it comes to owning a motor vehicle, insurance is now the largest component of the annual car registration fee paid by Victorian motorists. The registration collection agency, VicRoads, ostensibly builds and manages roads, delivers road safety initiatives and manages registration and licensing.[105] However, over half of the registration fee funds the work of the Transport Accident Commission (TAC). In 2018, this amounted to $521.40, or 64 per cent of the total $817.60 registration fee for a typical family car in the Melbourne metropolitan area.[106,107]

Most Victorians do not give much thought to their vehicle registration beyond its impact on the household budget. Some see the TAC expense in their bill and wonder where the money goes. This chapter describes how that contribution may one day save their life.

Pre-1970: In the beginning

In a 1992 essay chronicling the evolution of the TAC scheme, John Cain, Labor Premier of Victoria from 1982 to 1990, described the car insurance industry as almost as old as the car itself.[108] Following World War I, car insurance was optional and based on common law. This meant that those injured in motor vehicle accidents might get no compensation if a negligent driver was uninsured or without funds. Furthermore, any evidence of negligence on the part of the injured, if accepted in court, would result in no compensation being payable.[108]

The Motor Car Act 1939 saw the introduction of compulsory motor car insurance in Victoria. In contrast to Victoria's pioneering efforts in seat belts and other road safety measures, this occurred more than a decade after similar legislation had been enacted overseas, and four years after the smaller state of Tasmania had legislated compulsory insurance. This legislation, combined with a rise in motoring in the post-war years, led to a booming car insurance industry. By the early 1960s fifty government-authorised insurance companies were clamouring for business.[108]

However the excitement was not to last. Investor confidence faded over the following decade, as payouts were perceived by many to be overly generous, and as further legislative modifications were brought in to make the system fairer and more humane. Most notable of these was the *Wrongs (contributory negligence) Bill*, promoted by prominent Melbourne barrister John William (Jack) Galbally QC, who was a Labor member of Parliament in Victoria from 1949 to 1979.[109] The premise of this bill, as described by Galbally, was simple – to extend to land-based accidents the concept of contributory negligence, which had been part of maritime law since 1928:

> Whereas a shipowner whose vessel contributed to an
> accident recovers the true proportion of his loss, in the
> case of an accident on land, if a claimant is negligent to
> only a small degree, compared with the fault of the other
> party, he fails utterly . . . The harshness of the old common
> law position regarding contributory negligence was not
> so apparent in the days when a person took his occasional
> remedy against the coachman who ran him down in
> the streets of London; but to-day, with traffic accidents
> becoming, unfortunately, such a feature of our daily
> lives, a reform of this kind becomes urgent and overdue.
> (August 22 1951)[110]

Normally, an insurance company can offset higher expenditure by increasing premiums. However, because third party motor accident insurance was legislated, premium levels were subject to government control and therefore also to political considerations. The combined influence of contributory negligence and constrained premiums resulted in a dramatic withdrawal of companies offering compulsory third party car insurance.

By 1970, there were only two left standing – the State Insurance Office (SIO), which was underwritten by Government, and insurance offered by the Royal Automobile Club of Victoria (RACV).[108]

1970–1987: The need for insurance reform

Within the powerful human stories of *Declare War on 1034* was a lower profile but critical sub-plot; the financial cost of road trauma to the State. By late 1970, the rising number of road deaths had led to the government legislating rises in compulsory third party insurance premiums of 15 to 20 per cent. Further rises were forecast to stem the alarming deterioration in 1969–1970 in the ratio of claims paid to premiums obtained, from 102 to 194.2 per cent. That is, for every $100 contributed by motorists, $194 was being spent by the insurers.[111]

A key limitation of the insurance model at this time was the lag between incurring healthcare expenses and payment of insurance. Trauma care expenses accumulate from the moment of impact. In cases of moderate to severe injury, these expenses often extend for the rest of a patient's life. Ambulances, hospitals and other healthcare facilities providing trauma care had to carry these expenses for years as the litigation process proceeded through the courts.[55]

This problem was addressed in 1971 through the introduction of a 'partial no fault' system. The *Road Accident Hospital Accounts Committee* paid 70 per cent of an injured person's hospital bills before compensation matters had even been to court. This successful approach led to the establishment of the Motor Accident Board (MAB) in February 1974, by which time only one insurer, the SIO, remained. The MAB legislation enabled payment of medical expenses and income replacement until settlement of common

The Sun, Thursday, Dec. 17, 1970—Page 3

3RD PARTY MAY RISE: ROAD TOLL TO BLAME

By NEVILLE WILLMOTT

VICTORIAN motorists face a steep rise in compulsory third party insurance premiums.

The increase could be about $10—lifting private car premiums to more than $40 a year.

State Cabinet on Monday will discuss how much the premiums should rise.

The rise is certain, following a $13.4 million loss on third party insurance by the State Motor Car Insurance Office last financial year.

The insurance office says a big rise in third party claims is a direct result of the heavy road toll.

The Insurance Commissioner, Mr J. T. Inkster, said in a report to Parliament yesterday that the Statutory Premiums Committee had recommended increased third party rates.

This recommendation was based on the combined statistics of all authorised insurers in 1968-69.

Mr Inkster said: "As our office's 1969-70 results, comprising 41 per cent of the market, are so disastrous, still higher rates seem to be justified."

The NSW State insurance office lost $9.3 million last financial year, Mr Inkster said.

This occurred even though the NSW premium for a private vehicle was $40 compared with $31.65 in Victoria ($35.05 less $3.40 for surcharge and hospitals).

Mr Inkster said the loss on comprehensive insurance in 1969-70 was $387,373.

Claims up

The State Office increased comprehensive premiums by 15 to 20 per cent at the start of this month.

Mr Inkster said that the number of insured vehicles in 1969-70 rose by about 10 per cent, but the number of claims rose by 18 per cent.

"This will not cause surprise after reading of the heavy road toll," Mr Inkster said.

"Allied with the increase in incidence of accidents is their severity."

Mr Inkster said the claims ratio for third party insurance had deteriorated from 102 per cent to 194.2 per cent.

The claims ratio for comprehensive insurance deteriorated from 79.5 per cent to 86.8 per cent.

This was consistent with the experience of other motor insurers.

The deteriorated claims ratio on third party means the office pays out $194 for every $100 received in premiums.

Friday Blackest of year

TOMORROW — the Friday before Christmas — is the worst Friday for accidents in Victoria.

The Traffic Commission gave this warning yesterday.

The chairman, Mr J. G. Westland, said that more than twice the average number of injury accidents on Fridays during the year occurred on this day.

And driving hazards will multiply tomorrow afternoon when 776,000 State school pupils break up for the Christmas holidays.

The Victorian manager of the road safety division of the National Safety Council, Mr F. G. Harris, said history proved this was the worst time of the year for drivers.

He said 29 Victorians died on the roads in the corresponding week last year.

So far this week nine people have died.

● More reports, Page 17.

Page

Births, deaths	48-49
Theatres	54-57
Features	8, 9
Forum	34
Young Sun	36
Free insurance	36
Law list	37
Woman	38
TV	42
Crossword	43
Finance	44

Announcing the insurance premium hike
The Sun, December 17 1970, p. 3

law claims, which were managed by the SIO, and regardless of the outcome of these claims.[108]

These developments in Victoria were occurring within the context of a national discussion about compensation law. In the early 1970s, Gough Whitlam's Labor Government established a committee led by Owen Woodhouse to consider a no-fault personal injury compensation system. The Woodhouse Report, released in 1974, examined both the underlying philosophy and real-world operation of fault-based negligence action, including the risks associated with litigation, the potential for long delays, the negative influence of the system on rehabilitation care, and the costs.[112]

The Woodhouse Report concluded by recommending a national no-fault compensation and rehabilitation scheme for the injured and sick. Woodhouse had proposed a similar scheme for New Zealand in a separate 1967 report, and this was established in 1974. The Australian proposal was to be funded by a national two percent levy on salaries and wages, an excise tax on petrol, and consolidated revenue.[113]

The National Compensation Bill 1974 passed the Australian House of Representatives. However, doubts were raised in the Senate (the house of legislation review in the Australian Parliament) about the power of the Australian Parliament to abolish common law rights under the Australian Constitution. By the time the Bill had been re-drafted to address these issues (including with reference to the example of the Victorian MAB) and reintroduced in late 1975, the Whitlam Government had been spectacularly dismissed. Subsequent attempts by Whitlam to reintroduce the bill from Opposition were not supported by the Fraser Government.[113] The opportunity for a national insurance scheme therefore passed, and it was left to individual states to pursue their own.

Although ultimately stymied, the Woodhouse Report catalysed a national debate on compensation systems that was to continue for over a decade. The debate centred on the merits of fault vs. no-fault insurance and their underpinning legal and philosophical principles. The Woodhouse Report framed the issue in social, rather than legal terms, in which the central argument was that managing sickness and injury is a social responsibility of the whole community. Critics of the report claimed that it was unbalanced in its examination of the merits of fault vs. no-fault approaches; indeed, the terms of reference reflected a stated aim by the Federal Government to introduce a no-fault scheme.[112]

Proponents of fault-based systems drew upon over a century of tort law. (Tort law is a way in which the law can intervene between private individuals and make a ruling to correct a form of conduct or wrong.) Briefly, a fault-based system aims to address: (a) justice and morality (the idea that someone at fault should bear the loss of an injury that he or she causes to another person; (b) deterrence (fault deters careless or potentially dangerous conduct); and (c) compensation (an injured person receives benefits to compensate for the effect of the injury).[112] However the Woodhouse report painted a damning picture of how these principles play out in practice:

> . . . the fault system fails to accept the philosophy that is said
> to support it. It does nothing at all for the innocent victims
> of no-fault accidents. Compulsory insurance removes all
> personal responsibility from those who are supposed to bear
> the cost of fault accidents. It (the fault-based system) operates
> by shifting onto the broad shoulders of the general community

the losses of carefully selected plaintiffs (those whom lawyers choose to defend). And paradoxically, without the obligation of insurance, its attraction for both plaintiffs and defendants would disappear (cited by Robinson 1987).[112]

A thorough examination of the merits of these arguments is beyond the scope of this book. However, the effect of the fault vs. no-fault debate was to delay any substantial reforms, despite clear evidence that both motor accident and workers' compensation systems were floundering. By the 1980s the existing Victorian worker's compensation private insurance and common law model was in peril, with rising insurance costs and delays of up to two years before claims cases were heard.[114] Motor accident compensation was in the same position, but the Woodhouse experience, as well as similar examples at State level, had reduced Governments' appetite for change. As John Cain recounts:

> The liabilities represented by contingent claims continued to mount. The notion of starting a new system was not attractive to Government. The whole issue of compensation of injured parties had been seen as "a can of worms" for so long now and "band aid" ad-hoc solutions had been applied to keep the system limping along. Government continued in the same way right through the 70s.[108]

In 1982 the Victorian Government changed hands and John Cain from the Labor party became Premier. The incoming government identified the need to reform workers' and motor vehicle compensation, both of which shared a common challenge:

> . . . where you had a large pool of money, and an essentially adversary system, you had one group of people trying to get as

much from the pool as they could and another trying to pay as
little out of the pool as possible.[108]

Workers' compensation was considered the higher priority. Legislative
reforms by the Labor Cain Government revolving around prevention,
rehabilitation and compensation for workplace accidents culminated
in the creation of a new workers' compensation scheme, WorkCare,
on September 1, 1985.[114]

In 1984, the government formed a committee to reform motor
vehicle compensation. The challenges facing the existing model were
numerous, but primarily financial. In 1985–1986, for the first time
under the system established in 1974, total payouts were projected to
exceed income and the scheme would be unfunded by 116 per cent
in cash flow terms. This was the culmination of a number of factors,
including an eight per cent per annum increase in cost per common
law claim in the preceding five years and a large rise in soft-tissue
(whiplash) claims, from 10.3 per cent of minor injury claims in 1977
to 36.7 per cent in 1984–1985.[104,108] These rising costs underlined a
more subtle but equally important structural failure in the system: its
inability to adapt to healthcare trends over time. The MAB began in
an era when health outcomes following severe injury were generally
poor and there were no structures or resources in place to accommo-
date those that did survive:

> . . . if a paraplegic lived more than three years, after the
> accident without succumbing to some infection or something –
> it was the exception to the rule. Possibly people with head
> injuries survived better – but they were out of sight and out
> of mind; generally a hassle for people that had to look after
> them. But even amongst them, particularly the young ones,
> where did you accommodate them? There was no supported

accommodation, no facilities, people couldn't cope at home
so they put them in aged care facilities. So you had these
young people with head injuries stuck in with Alzheimer's and
dementia patients in aged care facilities. That was a problem.
And because the mortality rate from infection after significant
injury was so high, when we first designed the system for the
TAC, for many – that lifetime care truly meant what it said.
(John Bolitho, December 16 2014)[104]

Compounding these issues, evidence of fraud emerged and became public in September 1986. *The Age* newspaper reported systematic rorting involving lawyers and doctors specialising in false claims, large numbers of claims involving members of the same family or people from the same street, and staging of accidents. The advent of a new computerised system enabled better identification of fraudulent cases, which were reported to be costing the scheme at least one million dollars.

A further challenge, as faced earlier in the 1950s, was the political sensitivity of controlling compulsory motor vehicle insurance premiums, which were projected to have to almost double from $181 to $348 to cover the scheme's mounting liabilities.

Although the financial and political drivers of reform were clear, John Cain emphasised that there were important philosophical considerations driving the reform agenda:

We believed that there was a good case, as with WorkCare,
to be made out for moving to a concept that recognised
the preventative value of safety and the curative value of
rehabilitation, rather than just concentrating entirely on
compensation. We also took the view that revenue should be
weighted for risk and unsafe drivers with bad records should be

penalised accordingly. This was another way of saying that the community should exact some retribution against those who caused havoc on the roads. We took the view that, given a risk related premium, together with increased criminal penalties for poor safety performance, the removal of the notion of fault or blame from consideration of benefits was a logical step. It was a corollary of this that benefits should reflect the need of the injured party and that need should be met regardless of fault.[108]

A clear echo of the Woodhouse Report of 1974 (also commissioned by a Labor government), this led to a re-ignition of the fault vs. no fault debate. The legal fraternity fought vociferously to oppose the removal of common law rights. Advertising campaigns were funded by lawyers through the Law Institute of Victoria,[104] and their sophisticated political lobbying received extensive media coverage. According to Cain, and similar to *Declare War on 1034*, public debate helped create a political impetus for change:

> It was, in a sense, the old story – controversy ensures public attention and makes change easier to achieve.[108]

Himself a former lawyer and President of the Law Institute of Victoria, Cain was well positioned to recognise the pressure that was being brought to bear on political parties, for example through the Country Law Associations. When it became clear that a no-fault scheme would not pass the Parliament as a result of this lobbying, Cain responded by retaining a limited Common Law right, resulting in a hybrid fault / no fault scheme.[108]

> Effectively they (the legal fraternity) had the same argument twice and won twice. The first was on a national scale, the second locally. (John Bolitho, December 16 2014)[104]

The delicate issue of setting the insurance premium under the proposed scheme was framed around four principles: (1) Present day motorists should meet the costs of accidents rather than defer them to future generations; (2) The scheme should be managed on a full cost basis, measured against projected revenue and liabilities; (3) Premiums should reflect incidence of risk and claims experience; and (4) Additional revenue from criminal sanctions should be gathered from those who engage in anti-social road behaviour. The Government also proposed to fully fund the scheme for 10 years to enable cheaper premiums in its early years and promote equity between different generations of motorists.[108]

1987: The Transport Accident Commission

The Transport Accident Bill was introduced into the Victorian Parliament on December 5, 1986. The Attorney-General, Jim Kennan, argued that:

> It is necessary for all of us to recognise that the present scheme
> embodies inequities and inefficiencies that are no longer
> tolerable in a caring community.[115]

William Baxter from the opposition Liberal party articulated his party's agreement with the need for reform, but also emphasised its role in negotiating the retention of common law rights:

> There is no argument or dispute that the existing scheme
> needed radical surgery. It has blown out in cost for a number
> of reasons – one being fraud in both the no-fault area and the
> common-law area . . . The no-fault scheme proposed by the
> Government was inequitable and, although it might have been
> possible to run that scheme on the figures the Government

was quoting . . . it would have treated individuals as "meccano men" and worked entirely on the impairment table without taking any account of the relative significance of a particular injury to the individual.[115]

On January 1, 1987, the Motor Accident Board became the Transport Accident Commission; a Victorian Government owned, compulsory personal injury insurance scheme combining no-fault and common law benefits. On the surface, the hybrid fault / no-fault scheme was similar to the system it was replacing, in which the Motor Accident Board handled no-fault claims and the State Insurance Office defended and settled claims or damages actions brought against them. How did the TAC successfully address the problems that had rendered its parent schemes unviable?

Firstly, merging the MAB and SIO brought the system under one umbrella, breaking tension between the two organisations. Although the idea of separating fault and no-fault insurance seems administratively logical, the MAB and SIO's cultural (and geographical) separation were incompatible with the Cain Government's vision of a single entity that brought prevention, rehabilitation and compensation together. As described by John Bolitho, the SIO's primary focus was not on rehabilitation, but "buying their way out of future liability, incorporating it (rehabilitation) in the damages, close it off and get it off the books."[104] The MAB, in paying lifetime care and dealing with clients on a longer term basis, developed a greater awareness of the need to prevent and better manage road accidents.

> . . . trying to fuse the two cultures was a difficult challenge for
> the executives of the day. One was a caring, forward thinking,
> more empathetic group of people and the other people . . .
> were more adversarial-close-the-books. I think it took a long

time for the gentle culture to overtake the other . . . The
TAC . . . saw the nexus between the sooner you got people
rehabilitated, the sooner you can get them back to life, the
sooner you stop paying income support, the sooner they can
get on with their life and you get them off your back. (John
Bolitho, December 16 2014)[104]

This fusing of the 'hard head' of managing financial insurance risk
with the 'soft heart' of managing people who have been severely
injured has been driven in part by TAC being structured as an
'in-sourced' claims management provider. Today, there is simply no
capacity to bounce these functions between two organisations as
in the past. TAC claims agents deal directly with clients on a day-
to-day basis – sometimes face to face in their homes – rather than
through an intermediate agency. They often have to convey to their
clients decisions to withhold funding – for example, for a desired
medical procedure that is considered unjustifiable based upon expert
clinical opinion.

Second, although common law rights were retained, their scope
was substantially tightened. The right to common law action was only
given to those who suffered a 'serious injury' where the Commission
determined the degree of impairment to be 30 percent or more.
This eliminated claims for soft tissue and other minor injuries that
contributed to the financial demise of the previous scheme. 'Serious
injury' was defined in the statute, based upon a successful system in
Michigan, USA,[104] and covered serious long-term impairment or loss
of a body function, permanent serious disfigurement, severe long-
term mental / behavioural disturbance or disorder, or loss of a foetus:

. . . this is a matter on which it took a long time for consensus
to be reached at the various meetings that took place. It is

one of the most stringent definitions of serious injury in any
of the schemes we have examined . . . It should be plainly
understood that, although the common law avenue has been
retained, it has been so contained in the Bill that it will cut
out approximately 70 to 75 per cent of common law cases
and it will allow only those people who are suffering severe
disabilities to take that route. I do not believe it will generally
do justice to everyone . . . it is a matter of compromise to
come up with a scheme that covers the bulk of cases at a cost
the community can accept. (William Baxter, December 5
1986)[115]

Although a stringent definition of 'serious injury' was written into
the law, it has been subject to refinement and court interpretation
over the years. For example, the courts have debated whether a father
can also suffer from the loss of a foetus, although this was originally
intended to apply only to the mother. Similarly, the number of people
with moderate soft tissue and mental injuries accessing common law
is rising.[104] Therefore, although the 1986 legislation eliminated a
large proportion of common law claimants from the system, this area
has required close monitoring.

In fact the TAC also defined its difference to the preceding
schemes by being more responsive to change. The latest version of
the Transport Accident Act 1986, incorporating amendments as at
1 September 2015, lists over 85 amendments to the Bill, as foreshadowed by John Cain in 1992:

It should be recognised that legislation of this kind always
requires regular fine tuning . . . In the experience of the
fifties, sixties and seventies . . . Governments were too slow
to respond to trends, attitudes and court interpretations and

with the result the system got out of hand . . . The system has to be watched closely by those administering it and in turn the Government legislators must respond quickly where need is demonstrated.[108]

That the TAC remains in existence over 30 years after its inception, and still under the original 1986 Act of Parliament that created it, is the clearest indication of its success and financial viability. The workplace reforms of the same era, in contrast (although in essence now similar in structure to those originally proposed) were radically redesigned and renamed by successive governments.

The TAC's enduring success is testament to its unfaultering commitment to its dual roles – to reduce the incidence and cost of transport accidents, both of which were funded by premiums and income generated from wise investment.[55]

1990s: Where the money hits the road

The TAC consolidated existing community awareness of the horror of road trauma and its consequences, continuing the tradition established in *Declare War on 1034*. But as Victoria entered the 1990s, the formation of the TAC from the ashes of the collapsed MAB / SIO system also brought the financial cost of road trauma to public attention:

> . . . as the TAC evolved, with the cost of lifetime care and the cost of damages, people started to think about it in pure insurance terms . . . if you can stop the accident from happening, you are not incurring the liability . . . that's where the advertising evolved, and the booze buses, and all of that stuff. (John Bolitho, December 16 2014)[104]

John Cain and John Bolitho: Policy to last

By Melissa Marino

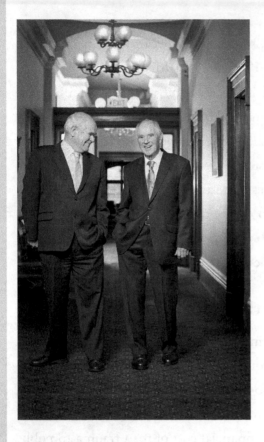

John Bolitho (left) and John Cain, May 2016

Image supplied by Coretext, taken by Eamon Gallagher

"No worthwhile reform is easy," says former Premier of Victoria John Cain, whose government was responsible for one of the most significant public health changes the state has ever seen. "But difficult achievements are a lot more satisfying and I am strongly of the view that what we got through Parliament was a first-class result – and a model for so many others around the world."

Cain oversaw the 1986 Transport Accident Bill. Although he'd been President of the Law Institute of Victoria, he met resistance from the legal fraternity, concerned the new system would water down common law rights and, notably, people's right to sue.

But despite opposition to the reform that would ultimately see the Transport Accident Commission (TAC) established, to Cain and senior counsel John Bolitho it was clear a change was required.

For Cain, there was no hiding that the system was struggling under ballooning costs and producing inconsistent outcomes. With insurance premiums on the rise, social and political impetuses for change were mounting.

"Certainly, the old system couldn't be allowed to continue," Cain says. "It had been limping along and the law was a real can of worms. Something had to be done and my job as Premier was to implement public policy that was in the best interests of the citizens of Victoria."

For Bolitho, as a partner with law firm Phillips Fox, advising the Government on content for the new act, it was clear those interests were not being served by the system. With the system being unable to meet the medical needs of victims, subject to fraud, congested with small claims, and costing too much in the process, he wanted the right to sue scrapped entirely and a no-fault system put in its place.

To say this position was unpopular in legal circles would be an understatement. "I'm still regarded as a traitor (to the legal profession) to this very day," says Bolitho, who has spent almost all his working life associated with the insurance industry, as TAC senior legal counsel, in his own practice and as an advisor to governments in the UK, Namibia and South Africa on compensation systems.

"If I had my way I would have no damages whatsoever," says the avid motorcyclist, who believes legal rights lost through replacing common law with a no-fault system are justified through benefits gained – benefits including a guaranteed level of care for all victims of road accidents.

Despite the continuing opposition of some of the participants in the system, Cain was able, as a member of a reforming government, to help shape a system acceptable to all political parties. Both sides of politics agreed to retaining common law rights to give plaintiffs a right to sue on a restricted basis within the new system.

"A dual system seemed to me to be a sensible way to go," he says. "You couldn't have politically got it through had we opted for a total no-fault system – society was not ready for it."

Negotiating this outcome is what the government did so well, says Bolitho. And what they achieved cannot be underestimated. "There is now this wonderful organisation (the TAC) that will look after you if you are injured on the road and it does so generously and in a financially responsible and viable way," he says. "And that is a great tribute to the Cain Government."

Cain had in fact had an interest in the notion of no-fault before he had even entered politics. He was fascinated by the relevant area of law – torts (or civil wrongs) – as a student, and his interest was further piqued as an articled clerk with John Galbally – who, as a Labor politician also happened to be a reformer of the preceding Motor Car Act (1939).

Soon after, as a young lawyer running his own practice, he witnessed inequities in the system first hand. "It was a bit of a lottery," says Cain. "The most deserving didn't always receive commensurate recognition in the damages they received."

By that time, as a member of the Law Institute Council, he was also involved in promoting legislation to fast-track payments to hospitals treating accident victims – payments often held-up for years as cases went through the courts.

Later, as Premier, he not only had the ability to act, but the benefit, he says, of being part of a particular political era where socially responsible, reforming policy was a priority, and to some degree, a public expectation.

The TAC came to fruition through a government that was "in reform/change mode," he says. This was a mode underpinned by the Labor Resource Centre, a collective of "left of centre" people including himself and future federal parliamentarians Brian Howe and Jenny Macklin. Established in the wake of the Whitlam Dismissal, it built a "reservoir of policy", including in Freedom Of Information, Work Cover and preventative health care, that would inform Labor's agenda for many years. "So many of those big reforms that I regard as being long overdue came out of that crucible of ideas," he says.

Among his own government's reforms, this one ranks "pretty high," he says. Even most of the sceptics soon came around to the merits of the legislation. "And that is because we put in place a satisfactory and fair system of compensation," he says. "The no-fault component – looking after injured people at a reasonable cost to the community – has been an unqualified success."

This awareness of financial costs was useful in softening the public to the enhanced road safety policing and penalties that accompanied the new TAC model. To fulfil its remit of preventing road accidents, the TAC used its revenue to directly fund Victoria Police through the development and purchase of equipment such as 'booze buses' (Chapter 1) and in more recent years through paying for enforcement activity that is over and above that which would normally be undertaken.[56]

In addition to funding prevention and enforcement, stable, ongoing TAC revenue also enabled investment in the considerable costs of caring for those who were severely injured on the road despite these preventative efforts. The rising costs of trauma care and the fact that many patients could not afford it themselves became a worldwide issue in the 1990s. In the USA alone, approximately 90 trauma centres closed towards the end of the 20th century. A survey of 313 US hospitals across 48 states published in 1994 revealed that 58 per cent of these reported that their trauma centres had serious financial problems and of those providing financial information, 69 per cent reported a loss.[116] Effective public policy responses to the same issues in Australia were needed. The birth of the TAC is an exemplar of such a public policy response. It was slow and difficult, but the system that was engineered provided a stable, sufficient ongoing source of revenue.

> . . . if the TAC wasn't here, all the trauma cost would fall
> on the Department of Health and the hospitals. If it was an
> additional burden on the system, I have no idea where we
> would find the funds. (John Bolitho, December 16 2014)[104]

> All of this engendered an environment in which improvements
> were felt possible in the trauma system . . . it's essential in
> the history of this to remember that the Motor Accident
> Board and the TAC realised the potential for this and were
> instrumental in funding some of the measures that have
> subsequently been introduced. (Chris Atkin, Surgeon,
> November 2011)[117]

Furthermore, the attachment of this revenue to an insurance system, for all the complexities and debates this involved, conferred a unique advantage through a financial impetus to optimise trauma care:

The TAC is a really good demonstration of why it works (the insurer framework). You actually take the long-term perspective of saying "Well I'm going to support this person as a result of their trauma". So I have an interest in (1) implementing it; (2) ensuring they get the best possible treatment in the world; and (3) they are rehabilitated as quickly as possible, to a level of independence. It's a pretty powerful framework, which we don't have in the rest of our public health system. (Rob Knowles, former Victorian Minister for Health, August 31 2012)[118]

. . . one of the great aspects of the Victorian State Trauma System is this inbuilt funding; where everyone – the community in particular – shares in the costs of the system; not unreasonably they have high expectations of the care that it delivers, and we constantly try and meet those expectations . . . as you reduce your road toll and injury rate, improve outcomes and get people back to work, and also there's a population increase, so your expenditure drops, your income increases and you're able to then invest in capital infrastructure. (Mark Fitzgerald, Trauma Specialist, November 2011)[119]

It is difficult to overestimate the impact of the Transport Accident Commission, and the refinements that have ensured its financial stability. The TAC addressed difficulties in the structure, function and financial viability of previous approaches to motor vehicle accident insurance that had persisted for almost a century and had seemed recalcitrant to both Federal and State-based attempts at reform.

Motor vehicle insurance faces substantial future global challenges. The advent of driverless cars and other crash avoidance technology has led experts in this area to predict that billions of dollars are going to be wiped off the car insurance business over the coming decade. This raises the potential problem of continuing to pay for the care of the injured in an environment where there is less insurance revenue to fund these expenses.[104]

Even in this context however, 1986 stands as a watershed moment in the Victorian compulsory motor vehicle insurance system. The clearest evidence for this is apparent in the case of one of the last Victorian citizens to be injured in the pre-TAC era – a six-year-old boy:

> He was run over . . . chasing a ball through an open gate and got cleaned up by a car. No one to sue, no damages. He was injured 22 days before the TAC Act came into being. So he was still a MAB client, but (fortunately) the MAB clients were absorbed into the TAC system. That fellow, they didn't want to release him from the children's hospital to their parents' care because they thought he would die there. Dr (withheld) from (withheld) hospital did a life expectancy thing for me, and it was an interesting read. I still remember reading it as if it was yesterday – if he survives to see his 10th birthday it would be a miracle.
>
> He has now got a teaching degree and a journalism degree, he has gone hang gliding, been on safari in Africa with his carers, and his life expectancy now – he'll probably make it to 56. He is now 30.
>
> I'm using this to illustrate that back in those days, no one was planning for the long term . . . (under the MAB) he

would be in diabolical trouble; his parents would have been in diabolical trouble. He had no one to sue. The lady who ran into him wasn't speeding – she did everything to avoid it (the accident) so he had no one to sue. His medical costs since are in the tens of millions of dollars. How could his parents have provided the 24-hour care for him? (John Bolitho, December 16 2014)[104]

The TAC's impact on the care this boy received, like tens of thousands after him, was immediate and life-changing.

Joe Calafiore: Beyond Insurance

By Melissa Marino

The Transport Accident Commission (TAC) is more than just Victoria's no-fault insurer. Funded through vehicle registrations, it supports those injured in car crashes as well as police enforcement and accident prevention through its push for safer cars, roads and drivers.

It has also been instrumental in the success of the VSTS supporting the development of vital infrastructure, from trauma databases to helipads.

The TAC's CEO Joe Calafiore speaks about its clients – people injured on Victoria's roads – as if they are personal friends. He knows their stories, how they were injured, their path to recovery and their prospects. He speaks of them with genuine passion.

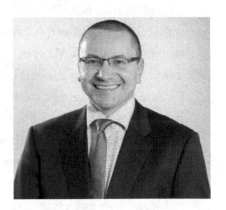

Joe Calafiore, CEO of the Victorian Transport Accident Commission, August 2015
Image supplied by Transport Accident Commission, taken by Ryan Gasparini

People like Anthony Bartl, the six-year old boy hit by a car in 1986 just as the TAC was being legislated. His catastrophic spinal injury left him able to move only his head, but with lifelong TAC and family support, the journalist and teacher is living a determinedly fulfilling life; flying microlight aircraft, snorkeling, sailing and travelling the world.

"We recently had Anthony in our building – he had made a documentary about his trip to Africa," says Calafiore. "He's the most amazing guy and he will live a long life and that is a beautiful thing."

The lifetime uncapped cover provided by the TAC – Victoria's world-leading monopoly social insurer for transport accident victims – is a feature that sets the scheme apart from others worldwide and in which Calafiore takes great pride.

Ensuring road victims achieve the best quality of life possible is its responsibility as a monopoly provider, Calafiore says, and this ideal is unashamedly a driving force of the TAC under his leadership.

Beyond its "principal duty to prevent", it puts the lives of clients at the centre, "making every conversation count", simplifying the complex processes and finding them the best solutions. And staff are invested in achieving these outcomes because the scheme is
"in-sourced" meaning they have direct contact with accident victims, he says.

This approach stems from the past, from something Calafiore remembers the TAC's founding father and former Victorian Premier John Cain saying at its inception that "stuck" with him: "The TAC is not supposed to be palliative care, it's supposed to be curative."

"The TAC is about much more than paying your bills. We are about rehabilitation, so what can we do to help you live an active life, an empowered life – a life of dignity."

A self-confessed history buff, Calafiore has an intimate understanding of the TAC's evolution, from its early emphasis on financial viability, to a shift in 2000 to client satisfaction, and now to optimising the quality of survivors' lives. "At TAC we aim to lead the world in social insurance and we are sticking our chin out to say 'The way we will measure our success or failure is in the health outcomes of our clients'," he says.

But to balance those results for its 45,000 clients, with a healthy bottom line, a certain level of pragmatism is required – and Calafiore is acutely aware he has a business to run.

"With the soft heart we've got to have a hard head so being authentic in our communication is important," he says. "We are managing $13 billion of assets and liabilities. The numbers are large – and performance only needs to deteriorate a little bit for the impact to be quite significant."

Ultimately healthier clients mean a healthier TAC, he says. And this is achieved through one of the "great geniuses" of the scheme that saw it built around three inextricably linked pillars: Prevention, Compensation and Rehabilitation.

"It's the virtuous circle," he says of the pillars that continue to define it and have led to improved awareness, enforcement, car and road safety, financial support and patient care. "To have prevention with compensation, it makes economic sense because as we invest in prevention less people get injured."

Funding and championing prevention strategies is one of the TAC's vital functions, he says, leading to innovative community and advertising safety campaigns as well as infrastructure such as Victoria Police's 'booze buses', improved vehicle technology and, via its major investment with VicRoads, safer roads.

Prevention is also the driver behind what Calafiore nominates as one of the TAC's most memorable campaigns 'How Safe is Your Car?', initiated under former CEO Stephen Grant, which invited consumers to 'rate' their vehicle's safety features online. Initially opposed by many manufacturers, it soon became a selling point for cars that met certain standards and led to the 'five-star' safety system actively used by industry today.

"We took an aggressive position and had to withstand a bit of pressure (from industry), but the market data showed it had an impact," he says.

Data also delivers an invaluable insight into the most effective treatments for optimal recovery through the TAC-supported Victorian State Trauma Registry, which monitors nearly all major trauma patients.

It also points to the best focus for future operations, including the billion-dollar Victorian Government 'Towards Zero' strategy – perhaps a somewhat audacious vision, but one made in response to surveys that suggested a certain level of complacency around road safety in the community.

Developed in partnership with VicRoads, the Victoria Police and the Department of Justice, and backed by Monash University Accident Research Centre (MUARC) research, it aims to reduce road trauma, with a focus on younger and older drivers, cyclists, motorcyclists, pedestrians and improving road infrastructure.

It's a big ambition, says Calafiore, but one rooted in a reformist and bold history that has always characterised the TAC, helped in no small part by bipartisan political support, and which has led to its success in reducing road trauma.

This boldness is also what attracted him, as a young ministerial adviser, to the organisation, which he joined in 2009 as corporate affairs manager while the TAC relocated to his hometown of Geelong.

"The TAC has always had a reformist mindset and the attitude 'Don't rest on your laurels', and that is because we have a monopoly and that's a privilege," he says. "We joke that we don't want to be the sleepy brown cardigans, so while we might have made some advances, we are always looking at 'What is better?' and 'What is next?'. It's a long game."

Chapter 3

MORTALITY

We speak for the dead to protect the living.

Ontario Coroners Motto – from
Thomas D'Arcy McGee MP
(1825–1868)[120]

By the early 1990s, the Victorian community had been exposed to over 20 years of public road safety campaigns, from *Declare War on 1034* in 1970 to the equally confronting Transport Accident Commission (TAC) campaigns of the late 1980s.

The formation of the TAC in 1987 had also addressed the vulnerabilities of previous motor accident insurance schemes, creating a stable financial platform upon which longer-term road injury initiatives could be built. This chapter tells the story of the Royal Australasian College of Surgeons (RACS) Road Trauma Committee from its inception in 1965 to its ground-breaking research to advance understanding of trauma care in the 1990s, which was central to the birth of the Victorian State Trauma System (VSTS).

The 1970s: A focus on road trauma prevention

The Royal Australasian College of Surgeons (RACS) Road Trauma Committee was first proposed in May 1965 at a meeting of Fellows in Sydney. RACS Fellows had become increasingly agitated with the extent of road trauma, which "destroyed more young men than wars" (Dr JL Tonge, quoted by Trinca, 1995).[5]

The Committee was formalised at a three-day seminar convened by RACS in 1969 and its initial remit was to survey road trauma incidence and injury, determine measures to prevent and relieve these burdens and identify organisations and strategies for applying these measures.[3]

To this end, in the 1970s the Committee focused on the development, implementation and evaluation of road safety legislative countermeasures. From the outset, it worked collaboratively with road safety authorities, motoring organisations, medical bodies and Government. A unifying principle of the Committee was referred to as 'the E.S.R. Hughes dictum' (Sir Edward Stuart Reginald Hughes was President of RACS from 1975–1978):

> Recommendations to control the road toll will be accepted
> if they are based on fact, scientific fact and only if they are
> practical and capable of implementation.[5]

The science underpinning the Committee's advocacy efforts was generated mainly through systematic recording of injury data from tens of thousands of road trauma patients. Use of this data, facilitated by legislation which made road trauma a 'notifiable disease', was pivotal to the seat belt and alcohol-related road trauma campaigns of that decade.[3]

The earliest example of such data – in fact, thought to be the first mass collection of detailed road trauma information in the world – was the Pattern of Injury Survey of Automobile Accidents, published by Peter Nelson and Gordon Trinca in 1974. The aims of the survey were to understand road accident injury patterns, improve treatment by examining delays in reaching hospital, document injury types, volumes and hospital length of stay, and provide recommendations to Government and other stakeholders regarding data collection, countermeasures and accident research. Between June 1971 and June 1973, reports on over 34,000 hospitalised patients and 1699 Coronial examinations were gathered.[121] The data collection used a four-page document filled out by the receiving hospital on arrival of every trauma patient, with their management and ultimate outcomes of their injuries recorded in the same form after hospital discharge or death.[117]

Key recommendations arising from this work concerned pedestrians, cyclists, motorcyclists, drink driving, rural road accidents, child restraint devices, improved vehicle design, funding of hospital staff, facilities, and the provision of public information.[122]

In 1975 Gordon Trinca also published in *The Medical Journal of Australia* the effects on road deaths and injuries of mandatory seat belt wearing.[48] Injury data was collected from almost 8000 individuals treated at or admitted to Preston and Northcote Community Hospital (PANCH) before and after the introduction of mandatory seat belt legislation in January 1971 (July 1970–December 1973). This analysis demonstrated that seat belts had reduced admission rates for car occupants and substantially reduced the incidence of severe head and facial injuries. However, this effect was not observed in children under eight years of age, reinforcing his recommendation about child restraints. Furthermore, side impact injuries were still severe and seat belt injuries were observed, leading to recommendations to improve side-impact protection in cars and seat belt design, respectively.[48] A second paper reinforced these findings by bringing together the PANCH and Pattern of Injury Survey data.[46]

Frank McDermott, a surgeon, was also active in promoting road safety countermeasures in the 1970s. He undertook surveys and analyses that built upon the above data, specifically through the blood alcohol test results from almost 43,000 road crash casualties (see Chapter 1) and a survey from June 1974 to August 1975 of 1320 consecutive road crash casualties admitted to The Alfred Hospital.[3,47,50] By the end of the 1970s, the RACS Road Trauma Committee was recognised for its role in road trauma prevention:

> The public certainly recognize the lead given by the College through its Road Trauma Committee in road safety countermeasures such as mandatory seat belt legislation and the identification of alcohol as a major factor in the cause of road crashes causing death and severe injuries. The College has played a major role in the introduction of blood alcohol analysis of adult crash victims attending hospital for treatment and random tests. (Trinca, 1977)[122]

Well into the 21st century, RACS continues to be a strong voice for road trauma prevention. For example, it regularly publishes and updates position papers addressing issues such as dangerous railway crossings, bicycle, motor cycle and vehicle safety, and licensing issues for both young and older drivers.[6,123]

The 1980s: Focus on road trauma care

Although data-driven prevention strategies were signature outputs in the 1970s, RACS had also been active in advancing trauma management during this period. This was mainly through seminars, education and standards-of-care initiatives, including a training syllabus for ambulance officers, and establishment of the Australian Resuscitation Council.[122] However by the late 1970s – perhaps following reflection on the injury data, as well as Fellows' frontline clinical experiences – the College signaled a shift in focus from trauma prevention to trauma management:

> The devastating effects of spinal paralysis, the suffering and disfigurement of victims of burns, the altered personality and diminished intellectual performance following head injuries, the loss of mobility and limited occupational potential due to limb loss and deformity, are striking examples of the need for effective rehabilitation services. The promotion of such services is one of the College's most important future roles. (Trinca, 1977)[122]

Similar views were held broadly in the medical profession and emergency services. Advances in trauma management included the establishment of Mobile Intensive Care Ambulances (MICA) in the early 1970s,[124] the introduction of specialised road accident rescue appliances in the early 1980s,[125] and the appointment of the first trauma surgeons to The Alfred Hospital in 1983.[117,126]

Despite these measures, management of road trauma remained relatively unsophisticated in the early 1980s – for example, head injury patients were strapped to trolleys to control their agitation, and in some cases were given a 'trial of life' overnight to determine their suitability for more intensive care and surgery.[119,127]

By the mid 1980s it had become clear that a new, more systems-based approach to trauma care was required. Surgical disciplines needed to be integrated to reflect the clinical complexity of injuries, and the high incidence of severe accidents in rural areas necessitated coordination of road and air ambulance services.

A number of events around Australia in the mid-to-late 1980s rallied groups around the concept of trauma systems. For example, in 1986 alone, a workshop conducted in Adelaide by the Neurosurgical Society of Australasia called for "better training, better communication, the organization of the trauma service at two levels and the use of medical retrieval teams."[5] American surgeon and trauma care specialist Howard Champion visited Australia, and his participation in conferences and the resulting collaborations were influential in driving reform.[128] Furthermore the New South Wales Road Trauma Committee held a seminar in Orange which led to the establishment of a Trauma Systems Committee in the NSW Department of Health.[128]

Subsequent activities reflected the dawn of a new era. Helicopter retrieval was established in 1986.[126] In 1988, The Advanced Trauma Life Support (ATLS) program, which had been running in the United State since 1978, was instigated in Australasia as the Emergency Management of Severe Trauma (EMST) Course, a course which "changed the clinical management of patients in the first hour or so after injury" (Atkin, 2011).[117] In 1989, the TAC funded Victoria's first Major Trauma Centre at The Alfred Hospital, which included a helipad to receive the most severely injured patients.[56]

The 1990s: Road Trauma systems evolve

The initiatives to improve trauma management in the 1970s and 1980s – including education and training, infrastructure services, helicopter retrieval, establishment of a Major Trauma Centre and the appointment of trauma surgeons – were all designed to reduce trauma mortality and morbidity. But how was the overall system performing? How could the success of these and other traumatic injury management initiatives be measured?

The year 1990 marked a new frontier in road trauma injury analysis, which arose from the seemingly simple question: "Could this death have been prevented?" For the next decade, answering this question became the central focus of the surgical, medical and forensic professions and – arguably more than any other singular concept – drove the design and implementation of the Victorian State Trauma System.

The concept itself – preventable mortality – was not actually new. Its origins were not even in the area of trauma. The New York Academy of Medicine's 1933 publication *Maternal Mortality in New York City: A Study of All Puerperal Deaths, 1930–1932*, is acknowledged as the first application of this idea.[129] And the roots of preventable mortality as applied to road trauma extend back to Columbus, Ohio, in 1955:

> Since the usual traffic accident affects more than one family,
> occurs in a public place, and is attended by law enforcement
> officers, it is usually highly publicized and there may be all
> manner of legal implications . . . The howling sirens, the
> flashing lights, the police cruiser, the questioning newsmen
> and the worried families, all help to magnify the situation,
> perhaps out of all proportion. It is with these thoughts in mind
> that a study was made of all the traffic injuries that visited the
> Mt. Carmel Hospital emergency room in the year 1953 . . .
>
> There were 30 deaths from motor vehicle accidents . . . in
> 21 patients, death occurred so rapidly, from such severe injuries,
> that no definitive treatment could be instituted. Analysis of

the hospital deaths was made to see if improved therapy could have lowered this mortality . . . Although abdominal injuries were infrequent, they were a major cause of death. Damage to a hollow or solid abdominal viscus must be repaired within a very few hours or a fatality will be the result.[130]

In subsequent decades, a number of further studies examined preventable mortality in trauma care. Collectively these showed deficiencies in care leading to poor outcomes where care organisation was haphazard, and, conversely, better care and fewer deaths where organized systems of trauma care had been established.[129]

The tipping point that brought the concept of preventable mortality to the attention of the Australian medical fraternity was publication in 1990 of the landmark US-based Major Trauma Outcome Study by Howard Champion and colleagues.[131] This study brought together data collected from 1982 to 1987 from 80,544 patients on trauma aetiology, injury severity and outcome across 139 hospitals. Over a third of cases were motor vehicle injuries. This data enabled development of outcome norms and therefore, identification of people who unexpectedly lived (defined as those who survived who had a predicted probability of survival of less than 50%); and people who unexpectedly died (those who did not survive who had a predicted probability of survival of greater than 50%). Statistical methods were used to generate indices at the institutional level that indicated the number of survivors or non-survivors per 100 patients that exceeded the expected numbers.

The development of such norms was a seminal moment for the trauma community in Australia.[127] Champion's study signalled a fundamental shift in focus from primary prevention to management of road trauma, because to this point road trauma incidence and outcomes data – the sort of data collected and published by Nelson, Trinca and McDermott in the 1970s – had been used primarily to develop, promote and implement road injury prevention measures:

> Australia had a very good reputation in the USA and UK and . . . we had never been involved in the clinical aspects of improved care, always the seat belts, helmets etc. so it seemed to me that I realised that I would be finishing in a while and so I wanted to go and do something clinically surgical rather than preventative. (Frank McDermott, June 6 2013)[44]

By illustrating how road trauma data could be used to identify and define treatment norms, best practices and outliers, Champion's study also highlighted that such data did not exist in Australia. Reflecting on a presentation by Champion at RACS in Melbourne in 1990, Frank McDermott observed that "we had no clue if any of these deaths that were occurring in Australia were actually preventable or not." (June 6 2013)[44]

Such data would have been unobtainable if not for coincidental developments in forensic medicine in Australia. During the 1980s, recognition of the importance of accurate forensic evidence was spawned by one of the most internationally prominent cases in Australian legal history – the Azaria Chamberlain case.

In August 1980, two-month-old Azaria Chamberlain was reported by her parents Lindy and Michael to have been taken from their camping tent in the Northern Territory (and presumably killed) by a wild dingo. Despite an initial inquest upholding their claim, a further investigation and trial led to Lindy Chamberlain being convicted of killing Azaria and sentenced to life imprisonment in 1982. Due to a combination of forensic inadequacies and the finding in 1986 of a piece of Azaria's clothing in an area heavily populated by dingoes,

Lindy Chamberlain was released from prison and the conviction was overturned.[132] This case, discussed and debated around dinner tables and at social gatherings across the country, drove a sustained argument for what was at the time a substantial investment in coronial services.[44]

In 1987, the Victorian Government led by Premier John Cain approved a new $25 million Victorian Institute of Forensic Medicine (VIFM). This was a response to existing autopsy facilities that were described by Stephen Cordner, VIFM's director for the next 25 years, as "a disgrace to the State of Victoria":

> . . . it was awful, the courtroom was there, you could hear the mortuary operating from the court. There was an open laneway where you could see bodies being transferred from funeral directors' vans into the back of the court. You look at those reports that came out of there now which were only 3–4 lines which were a disgrace; so significant as an autopsy be done [sic] and produce so little.[44]

Prior to this, forensic pathology was not a recognised specialty. Through the 1960s and 1970s the Victorian Government pathologist was a general medical practitioner, but by the 1980s this was considered unusual internationally.[44]

The appointment of Dr Cordner as VIFM's Founding Director cemented recognition of the professional role and practice of forensic pathology, which had been spearheaded by Cordner and other pathologists, and now supported financially by the Victorian Government. By the early 1990s, leading trauma surgeons including Ian McVey and Frank McDermott sensed an opportunity to harness the new forensic services to generate the preventable death data that was lacking in road trauma. As Dr Cordner recounted in 2013:

Ian McVey was founder of The Alfred Trauma Service and he was the first one through my door after we opened . . . there is a new institution that wants to make sure that it pays its dues, people have invested heavily and want it to be as valuable as it can be, so along comes Ian McVey who started the Trauma Centre . . . an extraordinary operator . . . he could get a Trauma Centre off the ground . . . he also ran the Medical Defence Association of Victoria and was President of the Victorian Branch of the Australian Medical Association, so he was an operator and a politician. (June 6 2013)[44]

The Consultative Committee on Road Traffic Fatalities (CCRTF)

In 1991, in his capacity as Chair of the Victorian Road Trauma Committee of the RACS, Frank McDermott met with Steven Cordner to discuss assessing the quality of trauma care. He outlined the problem of a lack of local data on preventable mortality and its relevance to optimising the quality of medical trauma services. They discussed how this could be addressed by undertaking autopsies on all victims of fatal road accidents to determine their cause of death and, with reference to records of their ambulance and hospital treatment, answer that critical question: "Could this death have been prevented?" Their agreement on this proposal connected those with expertise in treating the living with those whose profession is to determine and document how others died.

The result was the establishment in 1992 of the Consultative Committee on Road Traffic Fatalities (CCRTF) by the Victorian Road Trauma Committee of the Royal Australasian College of Surgeons and the Victorian Institute of Forensic Medicine.[44,126,133]

Chaired by Frank McDermott and Stephen Cordner, the CCRTF had two deceptively simple aims: (1) identify organisational and clinical errors in the management of medically treated road trauma fatalities; and (2) use this information to improve Victoria's trauma care system.[133]

The committee comprised 44 members: 37 from metropolitan public hospitals, three from the Victorian Institute of Forensic Medicine, three from Ambulance services, and one from a private hospital, plus a project manager. In all there were 25 surgeons (16 general surgeons, five neurosurgeons, three cardiothoracic surgeons and one orthopaedic surgeon), five intensivists, five emergency physicians, three forensic pathologists, three paramedics and three anaesthetists (Appendix 2 lists all CCRTF members).

The breadth of expertise within the CCRTF was designed to cover the full gamut of care from the moment the ambulance reached the patient to the time spent in the emergency ward, operating theatre and intensive care unit. Such breadth was unprecedented, even by comparison with the comparable initiatives undertaken in the United States, where audit committees didn't usually contain both neurosurgeons and orthopaedic surgeons, for example.[44]

Although the significance of freshly funded forensic services and the consent of forensic leadership to form the CCRTF cannot be underestimated, three further factors were arguably just as important to the success of the endeavour. First, although the newly minted infrastructure and personnel were in place, the actual work of the CCRTF required funding. Following lobbying by RACS and VIFM, the TAC provided $250,000 per year to the project.[44] As an insurance company paying for the care of patients, it wouldn't necessarily gain financially by funding an endeavour to reduce preventable deaths. That the TAC did fund it is credited in part to the influence of a TAC Board member who was also a TAC medical advisor, and who was therefore able to actively foster Board interest to improve medical management following road trauma. This, prior to the CCRTF, had led to direct TAC investment in trauma care infrastructure such as The Alfred Hospital's Trauma Centre and helipad in 1989.[134] Furthermore, surgeon Ian McVey had been instrumental in ensuring that the Medical Advisory Panel of the TAC reported directly to the Board, not a member of TAC staff:

> The Board didn't know what to do with this pesky committee
> asking for money; McVey knew that he needed to be a pain
> to the Board of the TAC to obtain funds. (Stephen Cordner,
> June 6 2013)[44]

The TAC funding employed research staff (a data manager and two research assistants)[135] and a senior nurse administrator, paid $100 per meeting to each attendee, and covered costs of catering, which was usually pizza.

Second, the CCRTF had statutory immunity to promote full and open discussions of quality issues under Section 139 of Victoria's Health Services Act 1988. This legislation was designed to ensure that confidential information generated by approved quality assurance bodies could not be disclosed to those outside of such bodies and was not admissible in court proceedings:

> The intent of s.139 of the Act is to provide statutory immunity
> protection for quality assurance bodies with a clinical focus
> that will facilitate improvements to health services and
> health care outcomes. It was designed to provide statutory

immunity in quite specific circumstances where a committee's emphasis will be upon the review of clinical practice or clinical competence.[136]

Having been declared a specified committee, the CCRTF was able to obtain autopsy information and cross-check this against medical records as an approved quality assurance body without the consent of either hospitals or the State Coroner:

> They couldn't actually stop it as we had our immunity. We got the records by virtue of the fact that the coroner required the records . . . It was all out of their hands, there was nothing they (regional hospitals) could do. It was all set up by Frank. Everyone was involved. Every element of the system was represented on the committee, so nobody could complain because they all had somebody there. (Stephen Cordner, June 6 2013)[44]

This is one reason why the work of the CCRTF was entirely focused on errors resulting in death, rather than errors resulting in non-fatal adverse medical consequences.[134] The Committee took care not to abuse this privilege:

> We never identified the single hospitals, [instead] we put them into groups, Rural or Metropolitan . . . (Frank McDermott, June 6 2013)[44]

Third, although statutory immunity rendered the approval of the Coroner a moot point, it was nonetheless important to the smooth running of the CCRTF. As Cordner explained:

> . . . we had access to the medical records by right. We had done the autopsy so we knew whether anything had been missed . . . We didn't need anybody's agreement that we could

do it [compare hospital and autopsy records]. The one thing we needed was that the Coroner allowed us to do it not knowing what we were up to. The Coroner was wanting the Coronial system to be as contributory and productive as it could be (but) not every Coroner thinks like that. Helen Stein did originally, then Graham Johnson, both of whom agreed to turn a blind eye (in a manner of speaking) to what Frank and I were doing . . . (June 6 2013)[44]

The Operations of the CCRTF

The CCRTF was established as a research project, with ethics approval from the VIFM. No ethics or other approvals were required from hospitals as records were accessed as part of the Coronial process.[137]

Answering the simple question of whether a road fatality could have been prevented was a complex task. For each Victorian road fatality, CCRTF research staff assembled a detailed account of all clinical observations and management using a data proforma containing over 1000 items.[135]

This catalogued every imaginable aspect of medical management from the point of injury onwards – the crash itself and mechanism of injury; results of initial assessment of the patient in the field; how the patient was managed and transported to hospital; all assessments, tests and interventions undertaken in the hospital; who was involved; whether the patient was transferred to another hospital and why; details of surgery and post-surgery care in the intensive care unit; care provided in the ward after discharge from intensive care; and finally, diagnosis of complications and cause of death.[137]

Injuries were coded using recognised injury scoring systems such as the Abbreviated Injury Scale and Injury Severity Score. Based on methods used in the United States, all of this information was used to establish a survival probability.[135]

All data was then sent to an expert CCRTF panellist for detailed review over a 1 to 2 week period. They would then present the case to the CCRTF, followed by a discussion between the various surgeons, emergency physicians, anaesthetists, intensive care doctors and paramedics who made up the committee.[138]

With reference to the Australian and American trauma treatment standards and manuals of the day, the CCRTF determined problems in trauma management for each case under five broad categories:

- system inadequacy
- error in treatment or management strategy
- error in technique
- error in diagnosis, and
- delay in diagnosis.

The Committee was then able to make a judgement on whether any of the identified problems were considered to have increased the probability of death or shortened life.[133,135]

Finally, the question of whether the death could have been prevented was answered by placing the case into one of three categories on the basis of a majority decision of the committee:

A preventable death was defined as one in which it was considered in retrospect with full knowledge of the clinical history and all injuries sustained that the chances of survival would have exceeded 75% with optimal treatment.

A potentially preventable death was defined as one in which it was considered in retrospect with full knowledge of the clinical history and all injuries sustained that the chances of survival would have been 25 to 75% had the patient received optimal treatment; i.e., had the patient been triaged effectively to a hospital with the appropriate facilities in minimum time and appropriate management promptly provided; and

A non-preventable death was defined as one in which it was considered in retrospect with full knowledge of the clinical history and all injuries sustained that the chances of survival with optimal management were less than 25%.[135]

The CCRTF was cognisant of the gravity of this process and its outcomes. All records were de-identified, and a statement was tabled at the commencement of each meeting invoking the statutory immunity underpinning the committee and the associated requirement of confidentiality of proceedings. As medical professionals themselves, committee members also appreciated that hindsight was not a privilege given to those on the front line:

> . . . committee's judgments had the advantage of retrospectivity
> with complete information on the clinical history and all injuries
> and complications, a review situation notably different from
> that of a treating team coping with a multiply injured patient.[135]

Considering the amount of data gathering, preparation and group deliberation required to categorise just one road death as 'preventable', 'potentially preventable' or 'nonpreventable', the collective work undertaken by the CCRTF is mind-boggling, especially given its appearance prior to the information technology revolution.

Two panels of 11 to 12 committee members met on alternate Friday nights – when the Victorian community was perhaps most energetically imbibing the alcohol that contributed to the road trauma epidemic – for approximately 90 minutes, 48 weeks of the year. Between 120 and 150 cases were reviewed each year, taking an average 45 minutes each, from 1992 until 2005–2006.[44]

Although the task of being on the CCRTF sounds onerous, reflections of CCRTF members convey a picture of collegiality, dedication to task and enjoyment of the process:

> . . . nothing had ever been done on this scale before . . . This was totally different from the many meetings I'd attended at The Alfred on mortality and complications; M&M meetings ('mortality and morbidity' meetings are routinely undertaken in hospitals to discuss and learn from adverse outcomes), where you'd have some complicated cases discussed and finished in 10 minutes. There was very little satisfaction in that. No one ever took decent records of how that would feed back onto the next case. It was all lost in words.
>
> . . . People said they enjoyed those meetings more than any other meetings they went to . . . Hardly anybody ever left the committee over the years . . . They learnt a lot. Everybody learnt a lot.
>
> . . . the people involved were very enthusiastic . . . Everybody knew that bad things were going on and people were obviously idealistic and keen for things to be improved . . . Maybe that was the reason, it wasn't just a cold dry sort of thing, there was a belief that these results would lead to an improved system and get better results than the ones we were getting. (Frank McDermott, June 6 2013)[44]

The CCRTF produced robust, trustworthy data not just due to the calibre of the membership and their sustained level of commitment, but also as a result of the strong underlying scientific approach. The method of determining preventable death represented best research practice, as it drew upon both medical records and autopsy findings.[129] It was also found to be internally reliable. Based on a sample of 60 fatalities independently examined by the two separate committee panels within the CCRTF, there was very high agreement on preventable death judgements both between and within the panels.[139] This meant that ultimately the findings of the CCRTF would be impossible to ignore.

The Findings of the CCRTF

The key finding of the CCRTF was that over a third of deaths audited were found to be either preventable or potentially preventable. The most striking feature of this finding was its consistency over time (Figure 1): "You would think that we'd reprinted the histogram year by year" (McDermott, 2011).[133]

The level of detail of the CCRTF process required to make preventable death determinations enabled in-depth interrogation of the frequency and nature of errors identified, and the extent to which they contributed to patient death. For example, in the first published audit of 137 fatalities from 1992 and 1993, 1012 individual errors were identified, primarily comprising errors of management (68%) and system inadequacies (21%). Errors spanned multiple points in the care pathway, most frequently in the emergency department (53%), during pre-hospital care (20%) and in the Intensive Care Unit (12%). (Figure 2)[135] Again, an almost identical and unchanging distribution was repeatedly observed.[140–142]

The CCRTF method enabled identification and description of specific errors in the five error categories. For example, management errors included inappropriate triage (that is, wrongly assessing severity of injury), inadequate fluid replacement or airway management, failure to successfully put in an intravenous line and diagnostic errors. Pre-hospital errors were predominantly system inadequacies,

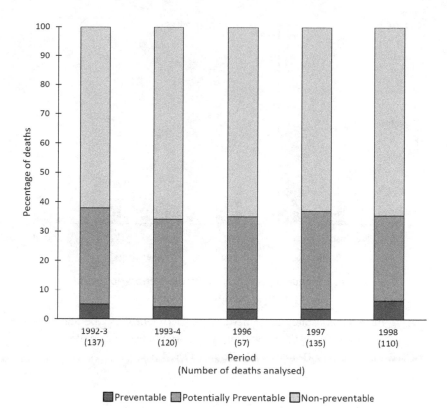

Figure 1: Proportion of preventable, potentially preventable and non-preventable
deaths among those audited by the CCRTF (1992–1998)
Derived from McDermott 2001, p. 110.[140]

such as spending too long at the accident scene or taking too long
to get there.[135]

More confronting than these relatively bureaucratic accounts of
errors at the group level were the individual descriptions of preventable deaths:

> A patient discharged home after a concussive head injury
> without a CT scan of the head followed by readmission six
> days later with a fatal subdural hematoma . . . Delays in the
> investigation, diagnosis, inter-hospital transfer, and dispatch

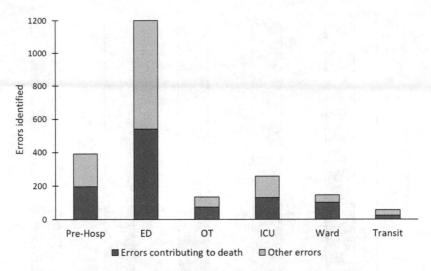

Figure 2: Frequency distribution of where errors occur and
their contribution to death

Key: Pre-Hosp. = Prehospital, ED = Emergency Department, OT = Operating Theatre,
ICU = Intensive Care Unit, Transit = transfer between care sites
Derived from McDermott 1996,[135] 1997[141]

> to the operating theatre of a patient with a thoracic aortic
> rupture . . . Death of a patient in a ward from an unobserved
> obstructed tracheostomy . . . (McDermott, 1996)[135]

The preventable death findings of the CCRTF were independently corroborated by a separate study led by Royal Melbourne Hospital surgeon Peter Danne, called the Major Trauma Management Study (MTMS).[143] It was an audit of management and outcome of 859 major trauma patients (including, but not limited to road trauma) presenting to five major Melbourne metropolitan and three rural hospitals between February 1992 and February 1993:

> . . . the percentage of potentially preventable or preventable
> deaths was 39.8 – almost exactly the same as the CCRTF . . .
> (Peter Danne, November 2011)[127]

The independence of this work from that of the CCRTF added to its impact:

> The MTMS was the other outcome study. Back in '91 I had handed a proposal to The Alfred people and was disappointed that they weren't interested in doing this together. Then I found the CCRTF being set up and I thought well hell, we'll do one too, and actually in the long run, little anguishes like that are good because that was fantastic that we had two studies. They had the same sort of outcomes . . . which backed each other up (Peter Danne, November 2011)[127]

Another highly significant finding of the CCRTF was that, based on examination of 257 fatalities between 1992 and 1994, significantly fewer problems and problems contributing to death were identified at the large metropolitan trauma centre compared to other hospitals and hospital groups.[144]

This underlined that where patients were treated was important. A system-wide remedy was required that could triage and optimally distribute patients to a hospital that could provide the care each needed.[135]

Key to this reorganisation, based on the comparatively good outcomes in the major trauma centre, was the idea that major trauma cases should bypass local hospitals in favour of 24-hour, specialised centres.[127,144] This had been demonstrated in large overseas studies, including the work of Champion and colleagues published in 1990 that spawned the CCRTF, as noted in 2011 by trauma surgeon Chris Atkin:

> The (United States) Major Trauma Outcome Study[131] was 80,000 patients plus . . . the (Victorian) Major Trauma Management Study . . . the CCRTF . . . all documented

the possibility that potentially preventable morbidity and mortality could be improved. From 1993 there were about 1200 severely injured patients per year, and by 1999 this had risen to somewhere between 1500 and 1800, depending on how you counted the figures. Among them clearly there were time-critical patients whose management and outcomes could be improved.[117]

After the CCRTF

Within five years of the establishment of the CCRTF it had become clear that Victoria had a seemingly intractable problem: one third of road trauma deaths were preventable or potentially preventable. The Committee had fulfilled its remit to demonstrate where improvements could be made to trauma care through carefully considered documentation of the failings within the trauma system.[134]

Reaction to the work of the CCRTF was mixed, and highlighted the sensitivities and difficulties involved in effectively communicating such findings. In an echo of the story of seat belts almost 30 years earlier, mobilising a response to the CCRTF's findings was not straightforward.

For example, the work of the CCRTF had made its way into the media, including a double-page spread in *The Age* newspaper on 29th July 1995 headlined "Patients die after errors at hospitals." It disclosed that "road accident victims are dying needlessly because of mistakes by medical staff, a secret report has found," and it was stark and uncompromising in conveying the CCRTF's conclusions: "the deaths of 30% of the victims who survive long enough to receive medical treatment are preventable."[145]

Certainly some readers were outraged, but overall there was minimal public backlash. Similarly, while the State's Chief Medical Officer was feeling the heat, reports to hospital CEOs and Medical Directors went unanswered.

> . . . he (the CMO) was perspiring as he heard about what we were doing and saying (Stephen Cordner, June 6 2013)[44]

> . . . the Department of Human Services and hospitals all knew what was going on but (we got) no response . . . It (the compelling evidence) built up, and to our horror, we were getting nowhere . . ." (Frank McDermott, June 6 2013)[44]

Responding to the intransigence of both the political and medical sectors, and declaring clearly its activist intentions, the CCRTF then decided to change strategy and engage other powerful groups within the medical establishment:

> . . . it seemed that ordinary communication was not enough and that if we wanted to have an impact we had to change our tactics. It seemed that we needed to formulate what should be done, and engage the thoracic society and neurosurgical society. So we undertook several working party meetings, in which we included their committee members, and we communicated with the societies. We came up with about 99 recommendations which we put in a report. (Frank McDermott, June 6 2013)[44]

That report,[138] published in 1997, became a sentinel document in international trauma care. It chronicles what was, and may still be, the longest-serving and most comprehensive preventable death audit ever undertaken. It presented the CCRTF's findings over seven years of review, and recommendations for how the identified gaps should be addressed. Beyond Victoria, the report provided a benchmark for the conduct of preventable death panel reviews, and informed the World Health Organization (WHO), the International Society for Surgery, and the International Association for Trauma Surgery and Intensive Care (IATSIC)'s Guidelines for Trauma Quality Improvement Programs.[146]

The 1990s had brought together a number of forces that drove the conception of the Victorian State Trauma System. First, there was a recognition that further advances in reducing the impact of road trauma needed not just focus on injury prevention but also on better treatment of injured patients. Second, the concept of preventable mortality rallied influential members of the medical and forensic professions to create a clear and consistent picture of the failings of trauma management in Victoria. Third, the nature of the problems warranted a systemic response.

Although frustrating for visionaries like Frank McDermott, the slow reaction to the work of the CCRTF is not entirely surprising. There had been enormous success in reducing road deaths from the activities of the preceding decades, including seat belts, breath testing and speed cameras. Between 1970 and 1994, the rate of road deaths had been reduced from 30.8 to 8.4 per 100,000 population, and from 8.1 to 1.4 per 10,000 registered vehicles.[124]

Perhaps the legislators and the community were also tired of reform; perhaps they thought they had done all they could.

But they hadn't.

> The State . . . continued to operate an ad-hoc trauma
> management approach in which trauma patients were generally
> delivered to the nearest emergency department and only 40%
> of major trauma patients [were] admitted to a major trauma

centre. It was increasingly recognised that a high percentage of deaths were preventable in patients who were still alive at the arrival of medical care. (Atkin, 2005)[124]

Finally, in 1997, a critical meeting was brokered with the Victorian State Minister for Health, Robert Knowles, and the Parliamentary Secretary for Health, Robert Doyle. Ten members of the CCRTF then presented their report.

Frank McDermott: Prevention and cure

By Melissa Marino

Trauma surgeon Professor Frank McDermott didn't set out to play a pivotal role in saving thousands of lives by dramatically reducing Victoria's road toll.

He first accepted an invitation from the Royal Australasian College of Surgeons' Road Trauma Committee chair and Professor of Surgery, Sir Edward Hughes, to analyse accident victim blood alcohol samples in the 1970s for the "numbers game" as he put it; and to apply his analytical skills.

"I wasn't looking at the social consequences at the time," he says. "But when we got the results we did, well, you have to sit up and take notice."

What that analysis – of the blood alcohol level in every road fatality – showed was that young-male drivers

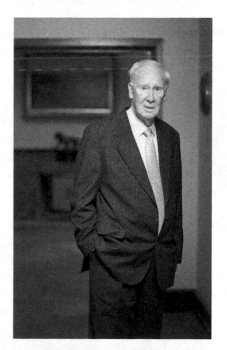

Frank McDermott, December 2015
Image supplied by Coretext, taken by Eamon Gallagher

were more at risk of crashing and being over the legal blood alcohol limit than those from all other demographics.

These findings lay the foundations for new laws in Victoria for zero blood alcohol levels for probationary drivers and set Frank's career on a course that would eventually see him determining key parameters of today's Victorian State Trauma System, which has become a model for trauma response and care around the world.

Indeed, he says, once the impact of his blood alcohol analysis became evident, he was motivated very much by a desire to create social change. "I wanted to work in this field because it was rewarding – it would have an impact on the community," he says.

As a young surgeon, it was never enough for Frank to confine his skills to the operating theatre. His inquiring mind always wanted to go further, to seek research opportunities to address the cause of illness or injury rather than just its outcomes.

"Research is where you learn new things, rather than just doing the routine," he says. "Diagnosing tonsillitis and prescribing penicillin is a bit dull. I needed something more to stimulate the mind – and this was shaping to be a fascinating journey."

This thirst for combining research with medical practice not only drew Frank to the Road Trauma Committee but soon saw him elected chair – a position he held for 14 years until his retirement in 1996.

As chair, one of his first acts was to investigate the safety of cyclists on the road. In surprise findings his research showed they were more at risk of serious head injury than motorcyclists. This motivated him to lead a campaign that resulted in world-first legislation for mandatory bike helmets in Victoria.

"It was a nice step forward," he says. "I drive around the streets now and see every cyclist – well most – wearing a helmet so I think it's been a very successful measure."

But while changes to blood alcohol content and bicycle helmet laws had saved many lives, for Frank and a team of likeminded health professionals, the next significant reduction in the road toll would require more than legislating to influence driver behaviour. Whatever the road rules, people would still break the law and take risks, and crashes would still occur.

What was required was a change to the system – a system, which, unlike people's behaviour, could be controlled.

Frank explains that in the early 1990s there was no definitive data in Victoria on whether road trauma victims could have been saved after their accident, had the response or the system been different.

So he set about filling the knowledge gap. Harnessing a trove of data newly available through the Victorian Institute of Forensic Medicine, with funding from the Traffic Accident Commission (TAC) and the enthusiasm of a team of 24 trauma front-liners jointly led by institute director Professor Stephen Cordner, Frank began to build the intelligence.

Despite the onerous workload he says he didn't have trouble convincing members of the Consultative Committee on Road Traffic Fatalities (CCRTF) to sacrifice every alternate Friday evening, analysing every post-accident road fatality in the state, to determine whether any of those deaths could have been prevented.

There was, he says, a real mood for change to reduce the road toll further, from the medical sector, politicians from both sides, and the community. And the work of the committee, he says, unequivocally underlined the need for that change.

In findings that surprised even him, they found that one third of deaths on Victorian roads were preventable or potentially preventable after the accident. In other words, those crash victims could have lived had the trauma response system been better.

This work enabled a clear case for dedicated trauma centres at three major city hospitals staffed by specialist trauma teams and serviced by an air wing and helipads for management of the most complex injuries, no matter where the accident occurred.

Their establishment helped halve the preventable death rate and improve outcomes for many more victims of trauma and his role in that, says Frank, was among his proudest achievements.

"Before this we weren't organised to manage trauma in a big way," he says. "It was like having a war but not having any battle stations or clearing houses or triage or anything. It was an empty territory really and was calling out to be done."

But like many people who are responsible for significant change in society Frank is modest about his role, reluctant to take any individual credit for any particular improvement to the road toll and the system. Rather he feels "lucky" that he was in a position contribute. "It's just part of life you know, that's all it is," he says. "You do what you can do."

Chapter 4

CHANGE

Mike Bloomberg, the mayor of New York, does
this party trick where he brings out a dollar bill
and then he snaps it and says: "It says on our
greenback, 'In God we trust' – and we do – the
rest of you bring data." And he's absolutely right.
Evidence-based public policy decisions are still
the best. And we had the data up front.

*(Robert Doyle, formerly Parliamentary Secretary for
Health in the Government of Victoria, speaking as
Melbourne Lord Mayor, August 31 2012)*[118]

The 1997 Consultative Committee for Road Traffic Fatalities (CCRTF)
Report was a call to action. It brought together hundreds of data
points on hundreds of cases, which had been catalogued, reviewed
and discussed at length by a panel of eminent trauma specialists first
convened five years earlier. This forensic, reliable documentation of
errors showed that one third of road deaths were either preventable
or potentially preventable. This chapter outlines the response to this
call to action, and the birth of the system that underpins road trauma
management to this day.

Call to action

Notwithstanding the gravity of the data itself, the CCRTF had a receptive audience. Robert Doyle, the then Parliamentary Secretary for Health, had a particular interest in ambulance services and pre-hospital training, to the point where he joined ambulances on night shifts to enhance his understanding of the sector.

And there were personal connections. Before entering politics Doyle was a school teacher, during which time he taught and tutored the daughter of Professor Frank McDermott, the co-chair and founder of the CCRTF. The pre-existing friendship made it comparatively easy for Doyle to seek out McDermott's counsel. Also, Doyle had drafted McDermott onto an Ambulance training taskforce some years earlier. And through Doyle, McDermott was able to connect the work of the CCRTF with the Victorian Health Minister at the time, Robert Knowles.[44]

The CCRTF catalogued deficiencies at every stage of the patient journey and showed that these problems were persistent. Life-support skills were lacking from the point of accident to the emergency department. It took too long to mobilise a response and transport a patient to hospital. There was no system for triage – identifying who should go where and how fast.[170] Transport between hospitals, like transport from the accident scene – was also slow. Emergency departments and hospitals not accustomed to major trauma made too many catastrophic diagnostic and treatment errors. And patients were dying because of deficiencies in care at all steps on the way – prehospital, emergency department, intensive care and surgical wards.[44,147]

The power of the CCRTF's message was matched by the credibility of the messenger. The evidence had been deliberated upon by a panel comprising eminent trauma professionals. Recommendations for action addressing the catalogue of identified errors were not the views of one person, but developed by consensus of the expert panel.[44] If this had been a court case with the Victorian healthcare system on trial, the case against it was watertight, a point underlined by Professor Chris Brook, a policymaker with extensive experience in health service redesign:

> . . . here's where things become interesting as to what
> makes good policy, because here you had a fairly strong
> basis of evidence; you had some very eminent and impressive
> people; and you had something which was of great interest
> to Government; something which they wanted at that time.
> (Brook, November 2011)[147]

The argument for system-wide redesign of trauma care was accepted almost immediately by both Doyle and Knowles, and it was clear that there was political will to respond.[44]

A key recommendation from the CCRTF, based upon the observation that fewer errors were made at trauma hospitals than at other metropolitan, regional and rural hospitals, was that road trauma patients with severe injuries should be immediately sent to specialised trauma centres, rather than the nearest hospital.

The idea of a limited number of major trauma centres is initially counter-intuitive; it posits that a severely injured patient should not go to the *nearest* hospital (for example, the local metropolitan or regional hospital), but instead be rapidly transported to a designated trauma centre potentially much further away. But what about the 'golden hour'? Don't you want to get an injured person to the nearest doctor as soon as possible?

The answer is usually no. A major trauma centre contains specialist equipment and infrastructure and a high concentration of staff with trauma care expertise, which is continually improved by exposure to a high volume of trauma patients (in turn a function of their designation as a trauma centre). Typically, a major trauma centre is also affiliated with a research-intensive university, meaning that staff regularly collaborate to build and publish knowledge drawn from their experience. For these reasons, patients do better in major trauma centres, compared to smaller, less-specialised hospitals.

The relationship between volume and outcome in trauma is well established in both civilian and military settings,[148] as well as in other areas of medicine such as cancer care.[149] It's not that smaller, local hospitals have inferior doctors, or that they don't do their best every single time they attend to a patient – it's to do with facilities and experience, with 'practice making perfect.' If too many major trauma centres exist, each will be seeing too few patients. Staff will then not have sufficient exposure, and the teams needed to function seamlessly in response to multiply injured patients, will not mature. Patient outcomes will be worse as a result. In Victoria, this was not a theoretical argument – the CCRTF data clearly showed that trauma outcomes were directly proportional to patient volumes across the various levels of the system. In short – when it comes to major trauma centres serving a population, less is more. As Robert Doyle noted, "the concentration of expertise argument is very difficult to resist." (August 31 2012)[118]

But health systems are not machines solely driven by academic data and argument, no matter how persuasive these may be. Health systems are hundreds of hospitals, medical centres and doctors' rooms, attended by thousands of sick and injured people on a daily basis. Each of these health services are run by clinicians and administrators with diverse and often strongly-held attitudes and beliefs, grounded in their own experience, motivations and interests. Funnelling cohorts of severely injured patients from previously dispersed parts of the Victorian health system to a small number of major trauma services was not an academic exercise – it carried real consequences for hospitals and other health services and the people who worked within them. This meant it also carried political risk.

Answering the call

Recognising the complexity of trauma system reform, Robert Doyle established a Ministerial Taskforce on Trauma and Emergency Services in July 1997. Its primary remit was to "advise on an appropriate trauma system structure and components for cohesive operation of a trauma system."[150]

The 34-member taskforce (Appendix 3) contained four members of the CCRTF: Christopher Atkin, Frank McDermott, Peter Morley and Jeffrey Rosenfeld. Nine working parties and subgroups (Appendix 4) covered role delineation, education, medical retrieval, neurosurgery, paediatrics, ambulance communications and system monitoring. The Taskforce also consulted widely with external specialist groups within and outside of Victoria (Appendix 5).[150]

Navigating the numerous political, logistical and other barriers to the revamping of Victoria's trauma system required, as Chair, every ounce of Robert Doyle's experience and diplomacy. As participants relate:

> It was a difficult task because there were arguments like
> there should be a major trauma centre at all the teaching

hospitals, there should be only one trauma centre, it should be (hospital X), or (hospital Y) and so on. And he handled all the conflicts of interest. There must have been about 80 people or more speaking with vested interests. He handled that very well. There was no nasty disagreement. Nobody was upset and thought they weren't represented. (Frank McDermott, June 6 2013)[44]

The Ministerial Task Force – when you look at that as a group, and imagine gathered in one place – I think Robert Doyle did particularly well in controlling the conversation that sometimes started to flow, and fortunately these were breakfast meetings, not after dinner meetings, which would have been I suspect positively physical. (Dr Marcus Kennedy, who was instrumental in establishing ambulance adult retrieval services under the VSTS, November 2011)[151]

As a parliamentarian he was able to use the sort of tactics that you use to curtail a debate. He would move things along rather than let there be a constant round robin of debate. (Chris Atkin, September 25 2013)[134]

The taskforce and working party met over 20 times, drawing upon the CCRTF, the Major Trauma Management Study (MTMS),[143] reports and advice from the subgroups and external specialists who worked closely with the taskforce as well as local, national and international publications, including academic publications from the 1980s and 1990s showing evidence of the success of tiered trauma systems in United States;[150] a 1993 Australian Report of the Working Party on Trauma Systems;[152] and a 1996 Victorian Government Metropolitan Health Care Services Plan, which foreshadowed a 'hub and spoke' system of specialised hospital centres, with routine procedures con-ducted in outer 'integrated care centres.'[153]

The resulting 182-page "Review of Trauma and Emergency Services Victoria 1999" report – known as the RoTES report[150] – became the blueprint for the Victorian State Trauma System.

In addition to reiterating the CCRTF findings, the RoTES report catalogued the development of trauma systems internationally and their emergence in Australia over the preceding decade. It was now seven years since the US Major Trauma Outcome Study had been published,[131] and data was starting to show substantial reductions in death rates at designated trauma centres in the United States. Nationally, the Australian National Road Trauma Advisory Council had released in 1993 a report recommending establishment of integrated state trauma systems[152] and efforts were underway in other states such as New South Wales and South Australia. By the time the RoTES report was published, its conclusions and recommendations generated little controversy.

What distinguished the RoTES report, though, was its depth and scope, and its focus on solutions tailored specifically to local problems. This would be no 'off-the-shelf' trauma system, instead it would be one ideally suited to the needs of Victorian patients, starting with what was already in place.

The 102 recommendations centred on the establishment of a formal system of trauma care that had three essential components: (1) the creation of a lead public agency with legal authority to establish and enforce policy; (2) designation of hospitals as trauma centres to provide 24-hour medical services; and (3) prehospital field protocols for identifying and managing critically injured patients who require direct transfer to a designated trauma hospital. The RoTES recommendations were built around features of successful trauma systems in 11 key areas:

1. Trauma System Structure – a coordinated system of Level I Major Trauma Services (MTS) in which there is concentration of trauma expertise, supported by urban, regional and rural health services that treat progressively less complex care to less severely injured people;[154]
2. System Organisation and Management – Committees and coordination units that develop trauma system policy, monitor system performance and address identified needs;
3. Triage and transfer protocols – a system for reliably assessing severity of trauma in the field and using this information to get the right patient to the right hospital in a timely manner;
4. Trauma Teams within MTS comprising surgeons, intensive care specialists, emergency physicians and other key trauma team personnel;
5. A Director of Trauma Services at all Major, Metropolitan, Regional Trauma Services and Urgent Care Services;
6. Communications infrastructure to enable efficient transfer of information, for example prehospital notification to the receiving hospital;
7. Retrieval and transfer staffing drawn from a roster to enable a suitable medical team to be mobilized and sent to the field where necessary, and the resources to support this;
8. Quality Management – establishment of a registry which collects data on processes and outcomes of care that is regularly audited and feeds into education and other quality improvement activities;
9. Education and Training – Collaboration between universities, specialist colleges and hospitals to deliver undergraduate, postgraduate and continuing training to support the system;
10. Research, Service and Technology Developments to identify and respond to trends and advances in telemedicine, information communication and technology systems for communication, diagnosis, and management; and
11. Funding – an ongoing investment strategy to prioritise key areas.[150]

In summary, the RoTES review brought together almost a century of learning about trauma care gathered from the theatres of war and those of hospitals and emergency departments around the world. This knowledge was viewed through the hard, disturbing and consistent data drawn from thousands of hours of meticulous documentation and analysis undertaken by the CCRTF, with the co-operation of the Victorian State Coroner. What was proposed was a set of unique solutions specifically designed for Victoria. It had the buy-in of all the medical professions. Its credibility and significance were beyond question:

> It's quite a sentinel document. It's very thorough, very detailed, and the greatest thing about it is that it's earnest and sincere. It's a sincere attempt to change public policy perception and outcomes. (Mark Fitzgerald, November 2011 – also see profile)[119]

> The Review of Trauma and Emergency Services or RoTES . . . has assumed somewhat biblical status and it is actually still a very important document. (Chris Brook, November 2011)[147]

> The review of Trauma and Emergency Services has been the sort of road map, the blueprint as to how the whole system would work, and I keep mine in a very safe place on the back seat of my car. (Surgeon Rodney Judson, November 2011)[155]

The Victorian State Trauma System

For all of the plaudits given to the RoTES report, the road to implementation of its recommendations was far from smooth. On September 18, 1999, the Victorian Government was unexpectedly voted out of office.

The 1999 Victorian State election had been expected to result in the return of the incumbent Coalition (conservative) government.

However, in "one of the most remarkable State elections of the last 50 years,"[156] support for the Government collapsed, especially in rural and regional areas of Victoria. The death of an independent (formally Coalition) Member of Parliament on the morning of the election heightened the drama, as a crucial supplementary election was required several weeks after polling day. Ultimately, 11 seats were lost by the Coalition to the incoming Labor Party – including that of the Health Minister, Rob Knowles – and Steve Bracks replaced Jeff Kennett as Premier of Victoria. Robert Doyle was re-elected to opposition and became the Opposition (Shadow) Health Minister.

> We had done the report in 1999 and five seconds later we were out. (Robert Doyle, August 31 2012)[118]

The RoTES report was one of the first given for consideration to the new Health Minister and Deputy Premier, John Thwaites. In his first weeks he was faced with a range of hot-button hospital issues spanning staff retention, governance and emergency department and critical care services – services that he later described as being "not only under great pressure but also under considerable media scrutiny."(November 2011)[157]

As in most Australian state elections, health was a contested issue in the 1999 campaign, and there were areas of considerable policy disagreement between the two major parties. For example, a planned privatisation of a major metropolitan hospital, the Austin, instigated by the outgoing Coalition Government, did not proceed under the new Labor Government.

However the RoTES report did not become a casualty of party politics, for two key reasons. The first was historical. As described in Chapter 1, the composition in 1967 of the very first Victorian Parliamentary Road Safety Committee was bipartisan. Both major political parties were equally vested in the seat belt law, from *Declare War on 1034* to the many other initiatives that followed. This discouraged populist responses to road safety because there was little or no political advantage to be gained from these.

> That bipartisanship enables politicians to take what can be quite a tough decision – as I'm sure it was when seatbelts were introduced and more rigorous drink driving provisions were introduced. (John Thwaites, November 2011)[157]

Secondly, the high credibility of the report itself meant that an incoming Health Minister who did not act on its recommendations would lose considerable political capital across a range of health professional groups.

> The fact that there were so many top experts that had been involved; it gave me the confidence that if the recommendations were implemented they'd not only be the right recommendations but there'd also be wide support for them across the health community. (John Thwaites, November 2011)[157]

This underlined another key factor that ultimately led to the successful adoption of the RoTES recommendations – they had the imprimatur of the community which was ultimately responsible for their implementation – the medical professions.

> . . . another important factor for those advising governments and politicians, to understand that it is a very tough and adversarial position you're in and if you can show that there is widespread support across the profession, across the health

industry, then politicians will grab it, because so much of what they're doing is trying to settle a fight between two parties. So if you have resolved the issues, solved the fight, you're likely to be successful. (John Thwaites, November 2011)[157]

After the Health Minister had accepted almost all the recommendations in the RoTES report, the process of launching the new Victorian State Trauma System (VSTS) was initiated. However, re-designing an emergency trauma system serving over four million people is not a perfect science. Winners and losers – real and perceived – are created.

> Although the experts had agreed, there was still an enormous process of change that was needing to be managed. There were a lot of people who were not totally comfortable with it. There were a lot of people who were nervous about the extent of change, and concerned about both the negatives and how they would work to implement the positives. (Marcus Kennedy, November 2011)[151]

The first and most obvious friction point was the process of designating hospitals to serve as the major trauma centres. The volume-outcome association suggests that the number of major trauma centres should be small. But how small? Victoria's population in 2000 was 4.7 million. The Royal Children's Hospital was designated as the paediatric major trauma centre for Victoria. However, opinion was divided on whether one or two adult trauma centres were required. Amid numerous political machinations and lobbying (much of which remains unwritten but tacitly acknowledged) there were some salient points – the initial willingness and capacity of the Royal Melbourne Hospital to serve as a major trauma centre; the broad geographical spread of metropolitan Melbourne;

and the idea "that having a little bit of competition between major trauma services would not be altogether a bad thing" (John Thwaites, November 2011).[157]

In addition to designating the major trauma services (MTS) as providers of definitive trauma care, other hospitals and facilities were designated within the system in various capacities according to location and capacity. Designations included:

- Metropolitan Trauma Services, whose role included stabilising major trauma patients prior to transfer to MTS and provision of definitive care to a limited number of trauma patients, where agreed by the MTS that transfer is not required; or
- Primary Injury Services, who either had limited resources or were in close proximity to a Metropolitan Trauma or MTS. These facilities would treat minor injuries only, and would be bypassed by ambulance to higher designated hospitals in cases of severe injury;
- Regional Trauma Service, providing a regional trauma management focus in major regional centres of Victoria with a similar role to Metropolitan Trauma Services; and
- Urgent Care Service, providing initial resuscitation and management prior to early transfer for major trauma patients in areas where higher levels of care are not available.[150]

The legislated ability to designate services meant that this was a formal process involving an explicit statement of organisational expectations, resources required, and desired outcomes. Away from the signature designation of Major Trauma Services, the process of designating all other Victorian hospitals, although less conspicuous, was equally fraught. A system needed to be in place to manage the triage process. Organisational commitment and cooperation needed to be garnered from hospitals to drive the changes required to reflect their different roles under the new system; roles that had the potential to be seen as a downgrading of their service.[151,157]

This process played out in various ways. Some hospitals embraced their new role in trauma care, and others felt that undue focus on trauma could worsen outcomes in other patient populations. Hospitals are not isolated silos; they are part of a system that is constantly reflecting on its performance and that of its components. There were tensions, and conversations about gains and losses. This reflected the system-wide nature of the reform and the scope of its impact on the day-to-day activities of a state-wide acute healthcare workforce.

It also highlighted that the corollary of concentration of expertise in trauma centres is dilution of expertise and experience elsewhere. A series of challenges in this context were outlined by Pat Standen, Trauma, Emergency and Critical Care Director of the Grampians Region (one of 5 rural health service regions in Victoria) in 2011. Smaller health services lost surgical services and operating theatres. This led to decreasing exposure to emergency care situations and, with this, the associated skills such as managing airways, fluids and the unconscious patient. This created difficulties in situations where these skills were called upon – for example when a patient was driven to a local Emergency Department in a private car, or when a patient in a non-trauma ward had a cardiac arrest. This also had implications for workforce retention, for example of nurses in rural health services.[158]

> There was significant change required . . . There was often
> up-skilling of staff; there were increased resources required
> in some places . . . less resources required in other places; and
> almost everywhere processes changed – about referral, about

communication, about transfer – and so again, in the usual situation of health – which is always under pressure – we obviously were asking people to change. So that was not a small ask in any respect. (Marcus Kennedy, November 2011)[151]

Of course, the CCRTF data clearly showed that outcomes were better with centralised trauma care. The difficulty was that this was mostly unseen by the rural hospitals that faced new roles in a statewide trauma system. To mitigate the risk of loss of emergency medicine skills, the RoTES report made 17 recommendations pertaining to education and training. However, addressing the 'de-skilling' effect of hospital designation, especially outside of metropolitan Melbourne, was to be an ongoing challenge for the VSTS. This was identified as a major area of focus in a 2009 review of the VSTS, *Trauma towards 2014: Review and future directions of the Victorian State Trauma System*:

> Education and training was considered an area for
> improvement, to address issues such as perceived deskilling
> of staff not working in a Major Trauma Service and having
> reduced exposure to patients with significant injury. Mindful
> of the health sector-wide workforce demands, particularly for
> nursing and medical staff, strengthening the trauma workforce
> through strategies to recruit and retain were identified as
> priorities.[159]

Stakeholders in the VSTS share this reflection and, more broadly, the need to ensure that hospitals at lower trauma designations, particularly outside of metropolitan areas, are not left behind:

> There are still opportunities for improvement, and some of
> these include in the area of education and training; the use
> of telemedicine; and stronger links with the Major Trauma
> Services. (Pat Standen, November 2011)[158]

I would have given a bit more thought to how you would
ensure that the upgrade of the outliers, because I think that's a
weakness. (Robert Knowles, August 31 2012)[118]

In Robert Doyle's reflections on the RoTES report he concedes that the language about centralisation was quite forceful and doesn't pay as much attention to the regionals and the second and third tiers as was intended in the Ministerial Taskforce meetings.[118]

Establishment of the VSTS represented the culmination of a journey that began with that first Victorian Parliamentary Road Safety Committee in 1967, continued through world-leading seat belt, speeding and drink driving legislation and campaigns, a complete overhaul of road accident insurance system, and then systematic analysis of the care received by injured patients. When unacceptable numbers of preventable deaths and deficiencies in care were revealed, an in-depth effort was mounted to optimise the post-crash response for Victorian road users. There were many champions, from many sectors. And the VSTS was their collective achievement. The task of implementation that lay ahead was no less significant.

We always think that the things that are evident to those that
are driving change will be accepted holus bolus by everybody
else. It's never the way, and active change management is
obviously part of what's necessary, particularly in something
as big as this. I think that we could have done more in terms
of inter-agency development and strategies for cooperation
and collaboration, and I think that we could have done more
in the space of education and capacity building in the non-
major trauma settings. And maybe they are some of the
challenges that still sit there for the future. (Marcus Kennedy,
November 2011)[151]

Although some attempts were made to sustain it, the CCRTF ceased soon after the inception of the VSTS. It had achieved its main goal of initiating major trauma system reform, and it had reached its limits in terms of what it could achieve through documentation of trauma deficiencies. Its focus on preventable deaths, that had proved such a powerful political lever, was itself limited in that it did not enable exploration of non-fatal adverse outcomes, and the increased effort necessary to do so was thought to be prohibitive. Instead, new vehicles and processes for collecting and analysing data about system performance were needed.[134] But the work of the CCRTF has left a lasting legacy. Even in today's information age, a world far more technically advanced than in the late 1990s, few major policy changes are supported by the volume, consistency and credibility of data that was produced by the CCRTF.

The winding down of the CCRTF doesn't mean preventable deaths panel reviews aren't important, and in fact they have been decentralised to become routine practice at the Major Trauma Services. But what was needed was a more sophisticated way of managing the change, monitoring its results and allowing the system to mature and evolve. With this in mind, the architects of the VSTS planned for a comprehensive, research-based monitoring system. This is the data we examine to find out whether the dilution of trauma skills in some parts of Victoria was offset by the concentration in the major trauma centres. This is the data that answers the key question:

Did it work?

Robert Doyle: Making government work

By Brad Collis

Robert Doyle's participation in the sweeping changes that eventuated in the creation of the Victorian State Trauma System was driven by a deep sense of unease. He perceived that the care injured Victorians were receiving was designed more to fit the needs of policymakers and healthcare providers than the needs of the patients themselves. Doyle concluded that, with a better system, many tragedies could be avoided.

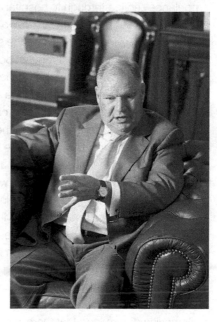

His involvement in the issue, as Parliamentary Secretary for Health, was at the instigation of the then Health Minister, Rob Knowles, who had been approached by the TAC with concerns that it, and consequently the injured people it was also supporting, might not be getting maximum benefit from its funding of the sole specialist trauma centre at The Alfred Hospital. The TAC

Robert Doyle, April 2017
Image supplied by Coretext, taken by Eamon Gallagher

had raised with Knowles a desire for some "competitive tension" in the system.

Robert Doyle – who after state politics became a long-serving Lord Mayor of Melbourne – was assigned to investigate. His first observation was the clear flaw in the number of decision-making steps and patient transfers between an accident and eventual treatment at The Alfred.

"For example if you had a serious head trauma in East Gippsland, the person would be treated locally, then a decision made that a higher level of medical intervention was needed, leading to a transfer to a district or base hospital, then invariably the same process of assessment and decisions leading to yet another transfer to The Alfred. Too often the time lost resulted in the patient arriving at the specialist centre too late."

For Robert Doyle two questions had to be answered: would it be better if patient delivery to a specialist trauma centre was the first call made? His answer, based on the advice of clinicians, was 'Yes'. The second question, therefore, was 'Would the State need a second specialist trauma centre to cope with this extra patient load?' and again the clear answer was 'Yes'.

But to make this happen Doyle knew he would need all parties – from the ambulance service through to hospital administrators – to be in agreement and for the health professionals, not politicians, to own and drive the changes. The key to achieving this would be the support of the clinicians, especially the surgeons, who were in the strongest position to counter any 'turf protection'.

Though a comparatively young politician, Doyle calculatingly initiated round-table breakfast meetings to ensure the many complex issues to be addressed and decisions to be made to radically change trauma care, were the day's first items of business for everyone. "And the time allocated was strictly adhered to so that everyone knew they were there for business."

Having decided there needed to be a second specialist trauma centre, Doyle recalls that Royal Melbourne Hospital was the only institution to initially show genuine enthusiasm: "There was nothing geographically pre-determined, so for example it could have been Monash Medical Centre (in the south-east) or the Austin Hospital (in the northern suburb of Heidelberg) but the Royal Melbourne was very keen and was also the preeminent neuro-surgical institution. It had some very impressive people including head of trauma at the time, Peter Danne. So it became apparent to me, very quickly, that Royal Melbourne was the right choice."

So having determined that there should be a second trauma centre and that it should be at the Royal Melbourne, Doyle then had his two champions: "I was able to say to The Alfred and to Royal Melbourne 'If you want to make this work it's not going to be politicians who will convince your colleagues about bringing people to these centres of excellence, it's got to be you guys and you are going to have to do that by supporting them both clinically and professionally.' They both made a commitment to do this."

However, Doyle says that Royal Melbourne coming on board was only the start . . . "just the lever" for other, sector-wide changes that had to be achieved before there could be a truly cohesive state-wide trauma system. "It wasn't enough to simply have another clinical centre of excellence to sit beside The Alfred," he says.

Through early discussions with surgical leaders like Andrew Kaye, Peter Danne and Frank McDermott, Doyle also articulated the need for research and advanced teaching to also be woven through the system; in particular upgrading ambulance officers to university-trained paramedics (later extended also to the Metropolitan Fire Brigade).

"Previously we used to put people on the road after just 12 weeks of training and it was as a part of assessing the adequacy of this that I started going out on the road with crews and seeing road trauma and the first response first-hand," Doyle recalls.

His objective, and that of his Ministerial Taskforce on Trauma and Emergency Services, was to create a seamless system "from the volunteer ambulance officer in country Victoria all the way through to the most senior neuro-surgeon at the Royal Melbourne or cardiac surgeon at The Alfred and everyone in between . . . hence the necessity of having all the players at the table; including district nursing, the ambulance service, the big institutions and universities. It was a bit unwieldy as a committee, but that was my job; to drive everyone towards an outcome."

Doyle attributes the ultimate success of this period to the support he gained from clinicians: "Personal and institutional rivalries and competition aside, when you asked the question 'Were we delivering the best patient outcomes?', their conclusion was 'No' and that we could do better. We had people sitting around that table who were more passionate about patient outcomes than their vested interests. It was inspiring."

Doyle also emphasises the importance of the process being led by the health professionals and not by a politician: "It was actually useful to be the dumbest person at the table and not have any expertise in this area because it meant that those who did have the expertise were the ones who had to get the job done."

And the job that was done was the development of what is today widely acknowledged as one of the most effective trauma systems in the world in terms of patient outcomes. It has been emulated elsewhere in Australia and internationally.

For Doyle personally he describes this result as the highlight of his expansive career in public office: "Of all the things I did in 15 years in Parliament and in the years since, this is what I take most pride in. It also came into effect after a bitterly contested State election. Change of government is an acrimonious time and the incoming Health Minister, John Thwaites, had been quite a combative Shadow Health Minister, but he nonetheless recognised the importance of the work that we had done, and he supported it fully. If it had been a politician-led exercise, perhaps it would have been different, but the Victorian State Trauma System, formally created in 2000, had been a sector-led response to a need for change."

Chapter 5

IMPACT

A beautiful thing.

(Peter Cameron on the State Trauma Registry;
Joe Calafiore on the TAC's role
in rehabilitation, 2017)

This book has charted three decades of response to road trauma – *Declare war on 1034* and the many world-first legislative changes that followed in the 1970s; the creation of the Victorian Transport Accident Commission to provide stable funding for road trauma in the 1980s; and the collection of data cataloguing how road deaths could have been prevented, in the 1990s.

By the year 2000, a complete overhaul of the state-wide trauma system had been introduced in the state of Victoria. The following year a comprehensive registry collecting data on patients' injuries, care and outcomes was in place. This chapter presents what the data told us about the system's impact more than a decade after establishment of the Victorian State Trauma System, and how the system works every day.

The risk of death following trauma had been halved in ten years

This finding took account of the effect of injury severity, age and whether or not there was a head injury (Figure 3).

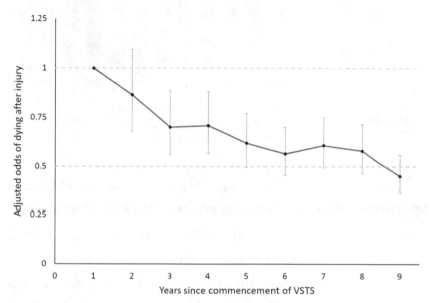

Figure 3: Trends in the odds of in-hospital death of major trauma patients adjusted for age, injury severity score (ISS), head injury and mechanism in the first nine years of the VSTS
Source: Reproduced from the Victorian Department of Health 2011[160]

The number and proportion of severely injured patients treated at major trauma centres increased dramatically

A significant goal of the VSTS was to deliver the patient to the necessary level of care in the shortest amount of time. For the most seriously injured patients, this meant straight to one of the state's three

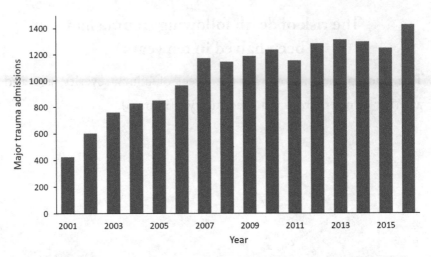

Figure 4: Major trauma admissions to The Alfred Trauma Service (2001–2013)
Source: Alfred Trauma Service

major trauma centres: The Alfred Hospital, The Royal Melbourne Hospital or the Royal Children's Hospital. Within a few years the proportion of seriously injured patients treated at a major trauma centre had increased from less than fifty percent to over 85 percent. Of course, the demands on the major trauma hospitals dramatically increased, as data from The Alfred shows (Figure 4). So significant was the effect on the hospital and its operating theatres that The Alfred built new elective surgery theatres to protect against trauma patients being overly disruptive of the other work a large comprehensive public hospital must do.

The quality of survival improved, but the medium and long-term burden of injury was large

Recovery from major trauma improved in the decade following introduction of the VSTS. Less than 1% were in a vegetative state – that is, unable to obey simple commands or communicate in any way. And it seemed that outcomes improved across the board, meaning that the system didn't save lives only for survivors to be extremely disabled and highly dependent for the long-term. Everyone involved, especially payers, welcomed the news of improved functional outcomes among survivors as well as improved rates of survival.

Despite these improvements, data also showed that, by the 12-month mark, still only one in five patients had recovered to their pre-injury level of function, only 74% were living independently, one third had not returned to work, and only 60% were pain-free.[161,162] So while significant progress had been made, a significant burden of ongoing disability had been uncovered (see Chapter 6).

The financial burden of road trauma care was reduced

Improved return to work and independent living were associated with reduced overall per-patient costs of injury. Societal costs also need to take into account the people who die, and people who survive but who live with disability. In 2010–2011, Belinda Gabbe from Monash University showed that the societal costs for each case of major road trauma were $630,000 less than in 2001–2002.[163]

Outcomes in Victoria were superior to those internationally

Studies showed that death rates were significantly lower in Victoria compared to England and Wales, which at that time did not have organised trauma systems.[164,165] This finding inspired change in England, as described by Professor Keith Willett in his position of Director for Acute Care for the National Health Service:

It's been my responsibility to implement regional trauma networks for major trauma across England. I am truly indebted to the work that's been done in Victoria, and I have been very grateful for the ability to be able to copy and to use many of the lessons that you have learned. I am sure I will not be alone in recognising the enormous contribution the Victorian State Trauma System has made to the improvement in care for trauma worldwide. (November 2011)[166]

In the US, it took ten years after trauma centres were designated for significant reductions in mortality to be apparent, whereas in Victoria such improvements were noted in less than half that time. This was probably due to the coordinated state-wide approach with simultaneous designation of hospitals and implementation of a new system for triage and transfer.[164,165]

How the system works

Teasing apart a complex system to examine its inner workings is a bit like pulling a clock apart and looking at all the cogwheels and springs – each component is important, but each depends critically on the other parts. Examining how the VSTS works is no different. Figure 5 summarises the VSTS in terms of its overarching and specific features.

The system kicks in from the moment of injury through **state-wide trauma triage and transfer protocols.** Ambulance Victoria responds to about 10,000 emergency cases per week, notified through a '000' emergency service hotline. With a 'Code 1' (lights and sirens) response, ambulances arrive at the scene within 15 minutes in three out of every four severe road trauma cases.[168] Ambulance paramedics

System-Wide Features
• **Stable, ongoing funding** of the system through the Victorian Transport Accident Commission (See Chapter 2) • **Victorian State Trauma Registry (VSTR):** for ongoing monitoring of injuries, response and outcomes, and enabling audit and quality assurance[174] • **State Trauma Committee:** provides advice to the Health Minister and the Department of Health on the Victorian State Trauma System (VSTS) by identifying systemic issues and exploring opportunities for improvement[175] • **Education and training:** driven by data from VSTR • **Research, service and technology developments**

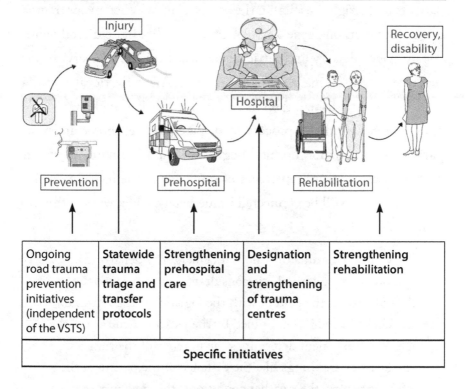

Figure 5: Overview of the Victorian State Trauma System (VSTS)

Adapted with permission from the British Journal of Surgery (Gruen 2012)[167]

access State Trauma System Pre-hospital Major Trauma Triage guidelines to determine whether a road accident victim meets one of three 'major trauma' criteria – abnormal vital signs (heart rate, breathing, blood pressure, level of consciousness); presence of an assumed or actual anatomic injury (for example fracture to major arm or leg bones, crush injury, penetrating injury); or a high-risk mechanism of injury (for example, ejection from a vehicle, car crash at over 60 kilometres per hour, fall from a height greater than three metres).[169]

Efficient triage[170] and patient transport is pivotal to getting trauma patients to the right hospital in the shortest time. When major trauma criteria are met, on-scene ambulance paramedics liaise directly with a state-wide advisory and retrieval service. Initially this service was separate to the trauma system, but in 2007 Adult Retrieval Victoria (ARV), was established. ARV is accessed through a single state-wide 1300 number, and the process of dispatching helicopter and preparing the destination hospital begins within 15 minutes in 95 per cent of cases. In over 80 per cent of cases one of the receiving major trauma services will be connected immediately, and always within 30 minutes.[171]

> The clinical coordinator, who is an emergency department, intensive care or anaesthetic consultant, has to balance the clinical need of the patient with the logistics of the retrieval. The clinical need is determined by the patient's acuity, and the acuity of the patient determines the urgency of the transfer. The logistics are things like the distance to the patient at the referring centre, the weather conditions, the crew mix that we have available, or the crew mix that is most appropriate for the retrieval – doctor, MICA paramedic or flight paramedic – and

the platform that we have available . . . fixed wing, rotary wing, or road. (Dr Charlotte Evans, Adult Retrieval Victoria consultant, November 2011)[172]

Victoria has the benefit that its relatively small geographic size makes most of its population reachable by specialised ambulance helicopters that have a range of about 150 kilometres. Since 1986 Ambulance Victoria has used helicopters, and there are now five helicopter bases in the state, providing rapid response and able to collect the patient at the roadside and deliver them straight to the helipad of a major trauma centre.

The **prehospital care** provided en route to definitive hospital care is among the best in the world. While many countries have doctors on-board ambulances for critically-ill patients, Victoria has invested in highly-skilled ambulance paramedics, robust protocols, excellent communications, and efficient transport. Ambulance Victoria, the statutory provider of pre-hospital emergency care and ambulance services for the State, is an agency of the Department of Health & Human Services, and was formed in 2008 following the merger of the Metropolitan Ambulance Service (MAS), Rural Ambulance Victoria (RAV), and the Alexandra District Ambulance Service (ADAS). In 2015–2016, Ambulance Victoria employed 3,438 paramedics and 578 specialist Mobile Intensive Care Ambulance (MICA) paramedics, and responded to 843,051 cases (including trauma and non-trauma).[168,173]

Paramedics are highly trained, holding an Advanced Diploma or higher, and their practical skills training and ongoing development are well structured and their career path highly professionalised. In comparison with many international jurisdictions, Victorian paramedics have particularly advanced qualifications and skills.

Notably, MICA paramedics are trained to perform Rapid Sequence Intubation (RSI) – a process of paralysing a patient and putting them on artificial respiration traditionally performed by anaesthetists in a hospital setting. A trial conducted by Professor Stephen Bernard, who is now senior medical advisor to Ambulance Victoria, found superior long-term outcomes in head-injured patients who had been treated with RSI prior to arrival at hospital, compared with those who were not.[174] In addition to RSI, MICA paramedics can perform a number of other potentially life-saving interventions before a major trauma patient has even reached the hospital, including needle chest decompression for possible tension pneumothorax, blood transfusions and clot stabilising medications for haemorrhage, and advanced life support for cardiac arrest, as well as intravenous fluids, sedation and pain relief.[124]

The decision to invest in highly skilled paramedics rather than medical staff for the prehospital care of the most critical patients stems back to 1971, when two paramedics and a doctor based at the Royal Melbourne Hospital undertook a three-month pilot during which they responded to 93 cases, mainly coronary care and road trauma patients. The Health Minister then officially commissioned MICA as a permanent 24-hour component of the ambulance service. The first MICA vehicle was a reconditioned Dodge 129 known as 'Car 208' that was previously the hospital clinic bus, newly fitted out with a stretcher, defibrillator and electrocardiography (ECG) machine. Ambulance officers chosen for MICA undertook a short coronary care course that had previously only been run for specialist nurses. Within a few years, the MICA unit was attending 250 cases a month and three other MICA units were established at The Alfred Hospital, Frankston Hospital and the Western General

Tony Walker: When time matters

By Melissa Merino

As a paramedic working in regional Victoria, Associate Professor Tony Walker saw his fair share of frontline trauma. Often first to the scene at car crashes, this meant dealing with distressing injuries including, at times, lungs punctured by broken ribs.

When a lung is punctured, air is expelled directly into the chest cavity, leading to a build-up of pressure that can compress the heart, reduce blood pressure and, in some cases, result in death.

This pressure can be released immediately by a swift piercing of the chest, but in those days, not all paramedics were permitted to perform the relatively simple, life-saving procedure. Only intensive care MICA-trained paramedics, like Walker, could administer it. And this put people at risk of succumbing to essentially a preventable death – particularly if the accident happened in a rural area.

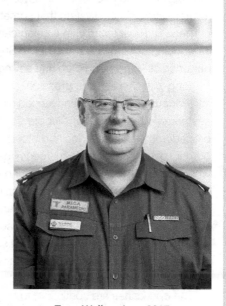

Tony Walker, June 2017
Image supplied by Tony Walker,
taken by Craig Sillitoe

"MICA paramedics were working mostly in Melbourne and big regional centres so if you were out of those areas the likelihood of getting those interventions was low," Walker says. "There were patients dying and not getting the best possible care because of where the trauma occurred."

But Walker, who by the late 1990s had worked his way up to a role overseeing clinical services with Rural Ambulance Victoria, would soon find himself in a position to remedy the situation.

Recruited with a number of his colleagues to the Consultative Committee on Road Traffic Fatalities (CCRTF), he was involved in work that laid the foundations for the VSTS – work that tellingly found one third of road deaths in the state were preventable or potentially preventable.

Among the reasons for this shortfall was the lack of skills among many rural paramedics for meeting the immediate needs of trauma victims. "Potentially preventable deaths were occurring because people didn't necessarily have the capabilities to intervene," he says. "In essence the CCRTF work created an awareness within the system that something needed to change."

These findings, along with a union campaign, led to the Government introducing training in Advanced Life Support for all paramedics – not just MICA paramedics – improving care and saving lives across Victoria.

Along with chest decompression, all paramedics could now deliver intravenous pain relief and advanced airway care. Further advances today see paramedics routinely helicoptered to accidents, performing at the scene procedures like ultrasounds and blood transfusions that are traditionally the domain of hospital-based emergency departments. "If you look back today to where we were 15 years ago there's no comparison," Walker says.

But the upskilling of paramedics was just one aspect of the reforms which now define the VSTS, in which Ambulance Victoria played a significant role: reforms to the system itself, including sending crash victims to specialist trauma hospitals instead of the nearest health service, and establishing Adult Retrieval Victoria (ARV) to coordinate the inter-hospital transfer of other patients to those trauma centres.

"The boundaries are continuing to be pushed and when you look at the number of trauma deaths reducing over time it is incredibly satisfying," says Walker, who, from the CCRTF, joined the State Trauma Committee, which was tasked with implementing the recommendations of the RoTES report to establish the VSTS and with advising successive Health Ministers on its ongoing operation, until he was appointed Ambulance Victoria CEO in 2016.

The success of the system, says Walker, has been in the willingness of those involved to refine and improve it based on "consistent evidence-based review" with patient outcomes the benchmark. Facilitating this approach is the database that records details and outcomes of trauma patients – the Victorian State Trauma Outcomes Registry, he says.

"The reality is once you measure something you can work to improve it and when collectively we started measuring outcomes, it gave us data to tell us how we were actually performing as a system," he says. "Prior to that we all worked in respective silos, but this told how we were tracking from our first response to hospital admission and subsequent treatment."

One insight in particular was responsible for a major rethink in pre-hospital care, he says. Before the data indicated otherwise, conventional wisdom said it was critical to get patients into a hospital setting within the first, or "golden", hour after their trauma.

But the registry data, since corroborated by peer reviewed clinical studies, showed it was more important to stabilise the patient at the scene before transporting them to a designated trauma hospital – even if it took longer.

"The evidence told us they did better because they were getting the right care immediately and their definitive treatment was provided in a centre that had all the capabilities to do it," he says.

And serendipitously, paramedics were equipped with the skills to deliver that immediate 'right' care through their advanced training, says Walker, who pays great credit to his Ambulance Victoria colleagues for embracing change. "New paramedics learn these skills at university but I'm still blown away by some of our older staff who, at the twilight of their careers, took on a complex training program because they wanted to make a difference – and they did," he says.

It's a willingness reflected in people through all levels of the system, from the paramedics, to the clinicians, bureaucrats and politicians who share a collective commitment to reduce the burden of trauma, Walker says.

"We have a standard of care that others are now trying emulate around the world and that's because there are no egos," he says. "When people come together around the trauma system it becomes a genuine conversation about 'How do we improve and how do we work together to do it?".

Hospital. Eventually it was decided paramedics were accomplished enough to respond without a doctor on board for even the most serious cases, and the modern MICA service was born.[173]

ARV not only directs the transfer, but also facilitates preparations at the receiving hospital by providing critical information. Before the VSTS, severely injured patients often arrived without warning, when surgeons were occupied in theatre, and other key personnel often unavailable immediately. A key part of the initial response after patient arrival was therefore assembling the team, which could take many precious minutes.

With advanced notification from ARV, and rosters of key personnel to be readily available when needed, the emergency department can assemble the team to be ready and waiting before the patient arrives. Furthermore, important information as shown in Figure 6

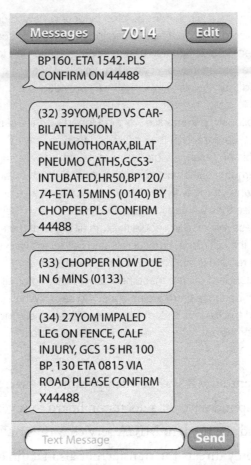

Figure 6: An example of prehospital notification of the critical details about road trauma and other cases being brought to a major trauma centre, enabling preparation by the receiving team.

that has been communicated before the patient arrives gives the team a sense of what might be needed, and opportunity to get equipment and operating theatres ready in advance.

Seriously injured patients are transported to high-volume **Major Trauma Services** providing concentrated trauma expertise through 24-hour trauma reception teams, on-site neurosurgery, cardiothoracic surgery, intensive care and other specialist resources.[124] As they are

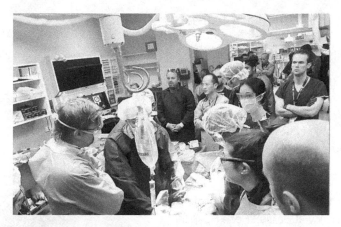

Major trauma resuscitations involve many people and
many concurrent urgent activities
Taken by and supplied by Mark Fitzgerald, 2018

rushed in from the helipad or the ambulance entrance, the reception
and resuscitation of such patients is highly protocolised, following
the 'airway, breathing, circulation' sequence familiar to first-aiders,
but with specialist medical and surgical expertise and many more
diagnostic and therapeutic tools. The initial response to acute time-
critical trauma patients is a unique process in medicine, in which the
time to take a history, do an examination, order a few tests and work
out what the problem is before initiating treatment is an unafford-
able luxury. Road trauma patients usually arrive with many possible
injuries, but little outward evidence of their exact nature, and what
is required to fix them. They are also often on a precipitous slope
towards early rapid death through inability of the lungs to provide
sufficient oxygen, lack of blood in the circulation to keep the cells
alive and functioning, or direct injury to the brain.

The treating team must identify and treat what is immediately life-
threatening – a blocked airway, a ruptured lung building up pressure

Mark Fitzgerald: Never standing still

By Melissa Merino

Pivotal in the path that led to Professor Mark Fitzgerald's commitment to improving the trauma system was a boy, who, critically injured in a country-Victorian car crash, died on his way to hospital.

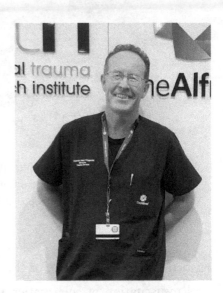

Mark Fitzgerald, October 2015
Image supplied by the National
Trauma Research Institute, taken
by Alan Mitchell Photography

It was 1998 and Fitzgerald, Director of Emergency at Ballarat Base Hospital in regional Victoria, was dispatched in a retrieval ambulance to the boy who had been injured in the crash near Ararat, some 90 kilometres away.

The boy was talking when Fitzgerald reached him, but had significant chest injuries and needed to get to Melbourne for surgery. But problems ensued as arrangements were wrangled for the boy's care and transport. A helicopter was dispatched, but it was too late.

"He arrested as we were coming in and died of a ruptured kidney," remembers Fitzgerald. "It was really frustrating because there were barriers to transferring patients and it was a bit hit and miss. There wasn't an organised system of care."

Plans, though, were afoot to introduce such a system and only a few days after the boy's death Fitzgerald received a fateful phone call asking if he would consider joining The Alfred Hospital to help establish its new Trauma Centre – a centre that would soon become central to the Victorian State Trauma System (VSTS).

Despite the move uprooting his family, he had little hesitation in accepting the role. "I thought 'Well, to change the system you actually have to go and change it'," he remembers. "There's no use complaining if you're given the opportunity to fix it up and make it more accessible."

As Director of Trauma Services at The Alfred, Fitzgerald has succeeded in that mission, advancing the Emergency Department (ED) in line with changes brought in with the new VSTS, centered around the hospital being designated as one of three – along with the Royal Melbourne and Royal Children's Hospitals – to receive major trauma cases by road or air from across the state.

This streamlined system, ensuring trauma patients are transferred expeditiously to centres equipped with the expertise to best treat them, aligned with other VSTS innovations such as improved communications between paramedics and the ED, to halve the death rate among trauma patients in a decade. Nowadays, says Fitzgerald, the Ararat boy would live.

But his hand in changing the system hadn't started with his move to The Alfred. As a long-time emergency physician and champion of trauma care, Fitzgerald was involved in training advances including the establishment of a dedicated College of Emergency Medicine, while also leading innovation in treatment through ultrasound and intubation. He was also a member of the Consultative Committee on Road Traffic Fatalities (CCRTF) whose recommendations informed the report that led to the VSTS.

And nor has his drive for continued improvement slowed. In 2015, his work on a Computer Assisted Decision Support System to reduce errors in trauma care and improve patient outcomes earned Fitzgerald an MD from Monash University.

The system, co-developed with, among others, Kon Mouzakis, then at Swinburne University, prompts medical and nursing staff to take particular action in real time through the first critical hour of care.

"A trauma team receiving the patient has to make a life-saving decision on average nearly once a minute," Fitzgerald says. "And without real time decision support only one in six severely injured patients get through the first 30 minutes without a significant error being made."

Operating in Victoria and around the world, the computerised system will now be enhanced with Google Glass technology in the form of eyeglasses that will not only record what the physician sees, but also feed them information and suggest treatment based on the data generated by the decision support system.

Fitzgerald's interest in improving trauma care stretches back to his childhood, and the influence of his physician uncle Jeff Fitzgerald who himself lost a son in a road accident, and helped establish the Preston and Northcote Community Hospital (PANCH) – one of the first to have a focus on accidents.

This is the same uncle responsible for introducing Fitzgerald to a concept that would define his career: the power of medical innovation.

In 1944 and suffering from rheumatic fever, his medical student uncle was the beneficiary of a new drug called Penicillin – his doctors sourcing just one dose from US Marines medical staff, who in the aftermath of the World War Two Guadalcanal Campaign, were camped out at Melbourne's famous sporting ground, the MCG.

Distilling subsequent doses from his urine, his uncle was able to extract enough of the drug for it to work. "It was sort of like gold and he recovered, which was quite spectacular," Fitzgerald says.

The impression of the incident was long-lasting for Fitzgerald (who harbours a keen interest in military history).

With an expensive university degree out of the question, Fitzgerald was on the precipice of enlisting in the Australian Army to serve in Vietnam when, in 1972, Prime Minister Gough Whitlam was elected, withdrew the troops and made university education free. Almost overnight, Fitzgerald's biggest dilemma then became whether to study medicine or art. Should he follow in his much-admired uncle's footsteps – or pursue his passion for art history and portraiture?

"My father said 'It's very difficult to make a living as an artist but if you do medicine you can always paint'," Fitzgerald remembers. And it was true.

Fitzgerald, who supported his medical degree by illustrating children's books, still does paint, his work adorning the walls of the National Trauma Research Institute where he is also Director, integrating research, medical technologies and trauma system development to improve care of the injured.

"It was the best advice he ever gave me," he said of his father's careers counselling. And thousands would agree.

in the chest, small amounts of bleeding compressing the brain or preventing the heart from pumping properly, or massive bleeding from a ruptured organ causing haemorrhagic shock.

Much research has gone into optimising clinical emergency teams for such care. The resuscitation cubicle can be a crowded place, with emergency physicians, surgeons, intensive care specialists, paramedics, nurses and other allied health clinicians all surrounding a patient whose status and vital signs change by the minute, or even more frequently. Keys to successful trauma response teams include having a dedicated experienced team leader, role delineation with identifying uniforms, and crowd control. To aid decision-making in this complex, chaotic and error-prone environment the WHO has recently developed a paper-based Trauma Care Checklist. Long before that, however, the Alfred Emergency Department had shown in a study of over 1000 trauma resuscitations that computerised decision support can also reduce errors and improve clinical outcomes, and the Trauma Reception and Resuscitation tool is now used for most cases.[175]

Following Emergency Department care, major trauma patients are admitted to hospital. For the most severely injured, this will mean a period of time in the Intensive Care Unit, which offers life-support, ongoing treatment, continuous monitoring and one-on-one nursing. The patient may need further surgery, and specialist support for organ functions, nutrition, bowel and bladder function, and skin care. Visiting family members, who are often coming to terms with the gravity of a loved one's injuries, are also provided a range of supports.

Once weaned off life-support, and recovering to the point that intensive care is no longer required, patients are transferred to a hospital ward. Here healing of tissues continues, supported by ongoing medical and nursing care, and often involving further surgery. Rehabilitation commences on the ward, and sometimes even in the ICU, involving a range of allied health professionals including physiotherapists, occupational therapists, psychologists, social workers, nursing staff and other specialists. A shared awareness of each patients' particular medical, physical, mental, emotional and social needs is fostered through collaborative multidisciplinary teams. From the moment that emergency needs are met the recovery process begins, aiming to restore the patient to his or her pre-injured state and, if that is likely to be impossible, to optimising function, independence and quality of life.

When patients no longer need inpatient hospital management they can be discharged home or to a specialist inpatient rehabilitation or long-term care facility. The needs of each patient and the initial recovery goals are determined by a specialist team, and a discharge plan is made. Some physical or cognitive impairments may be permanent and require long-term physical re-training and adaptation, home modifications, and training and support for family members. Patients with significant brain injury may need to relearn cognitive, behavioural and social skills. A range of inpatient and community-based rehabilitation and support services across the State identify and address ongoing medical, physical, mental and emotional needs, support carers of the injured and promote social reintegration and return to employment.[176]

All expenses on this long, costly and often arduous journey are met by the TAC – by the money that all motorists pay when they register a vehicle for use in Victoria.

Measuring system performance: The Victorian State Trauma Registry

Feedback drives humans. As children, we are rewarded and punished for our behaviour at home, and later for our performance (and behaviour) at school. As adults, the feedback loops multiply and extend, from everyday tasks of life – driving, cooking, exercising – to the work we do. The tick of the building inspector; the kick on goal; the hotel review; the often dreaded 'annual performance development meeting.' Validation motivates; criticism confronts and asks for, or demands, a change in performance. As the 20th century has unfolded, access to data has been exponentially increasing, challenging our ability to identify, grasp and use meaningful data without getting distracted by reams of extraneous information.

Feedback at an individual level is seen daily and easy to grasp. But how do you measure performance of a system? The Victorian State Trauma Registry was born at the turn of the century – less than two decades ago, but aeons ago in the context of technology and information dissemination. In the year 2000, the widespread growth of the internet had begun less than 10 years previously, and smartphones were more than five years away. But like the work of the CCRTF, the registry was built not on shiny technology but on the one fundamental of feedback – data.

Data to create the VSTS

The CCRTF had painstakingly catalogued deaths on the roads and examined their preventability, leading to the formation of the Ministerial Taskforce on Trauma and Emergency Services. Among many discussion papers tabled at over 20 meetings of the Taskforce were research studies of Peter Cameron (see profile) and his colleagues which mapped out trauma in the State of Victoria – how frequent it was, the cause, location, types of injuries, and outcomes. It was known from international literature, particularly from the United States, that trauma systems with centralised major trauma services led to better outcomes. But there was no data to inform how such systems would play out in Australia – a country with vastly different geography, population size and, therefore, injury distribution. This research – a world first regional dataset of major trauma – created this data by cataloguing almost 3000 cases of trauma in Victoria over a one-year period.

Such data was critical in informing the design of the VSTS. For example, it showed that serious abdominal injuries were uncommon, and spread across more than 25 hospitals, meaning that most individual surgeons would, at best, see only a few cases per year – and well below the number of cases required to have specific expertise in dealing with such injuries. It showed that there was a high enough volume of major trauma cases to justify having two adult Major Trauma

Services – a decision that has built critical redundancy into the system, for example in the event of power blackouts, computer system failure or a natural disaster affecting one, but not both centres. It showed that the two trauma centres should be in the Melbourne metropolitan area in order to maximise geographical coverage of the State.

These are all concrete examples, built on hard figures. But there was also the less tangible effect of the existence of the data itself. There were over 30 people involved in the Ministerial Taskforce, "all thinking the same but different" (Peter Cameron, December 2 2016).[177] Everyone had a stake in the outcome, but without the rallying point of data (and Robert Doyle) the conversation could easily have been steered towards the views and individual biases of any one of those individuals.

The registry was established in 2001 and had a number of critical features. First, like the wider trauma system, it had a stable financial platform in the TAC, whose substantial investment in the VSTS was conditional upon action by the Victorian Department of Health on all the RoTES recommendations, *including monitoring of the system*. This reflected a strong commitment by the TAC to maximising health outcomes following road trauma – an expansion of the remit of an organisation that (rightly) also has to ensure that insurance premiums are kept under control (see Joe Calafiore profile). The TAC saw that measuring system performance was pivotal to realising this ambition.

Second, the registry was run by Monash University, at the instigation of Professor John McNeil, head of the university's Department of Epidemiology and Preventive Medicine. Governments monitor systems and collect data across all of their programs and services, but housing this monitoring within a university was not a trivial administrative detail; it exposed the registry to ethical oversight by every participating hospital and health service. Research ethics review involves examination of all aspects of a proposed project, with an emphasis on the balance between risks to research participants and benefits to both themselves and the wider community. It is conducted by central ethics committees based at universities, as well as committees at other sites where the research is taking place – in this case the entire Victorian hospital and rehabilitation system. About nine out of 10 health services readily signed up to the registry via their hospital ethics committees, but there was resistance from some quarters. Was this a giant research experiment to see if trauma systems worked? A critical dashboard for managing a complex system? Or both?

This brings us to the third critical feature of the registry, a feature which exercised the minds of ethics committees. The registry was an 'opt out' registry – that is, all patients who experienced major trauma in Victoria were automatically enrolled in the registry, and given an opportunity to opt out at a later date. Intuitively, this makes sense – imagine a researcher with a clipboard trying to get a signature of an unconscious patient on an ambulance trolley, or trying to obtain consent through their distressed relative. History has shown that the vast majority of patients are comfortable with the 'opt out' concept and clearly see the value of the registry in which they have to participate (patients are interviewed periodically by telephone to collect ongoing data on their health and functional status); less than one per cent of patients remove themselves from the registry. But the ethics of automatic patient enrolment in a trauma registry – amplified by the politics of telegraphing the resulting data from every hospital in the state to a single university-based project – took years to fully resolve. It was 2005 before every hospital in Victoria was reporting their cases to the registry.[126]

Data to justify and embed the change

The registry collects high-quality data from all cases of major trauma in Victoria, in all hospital and health care facilities. If you were to experience major trauma in Victoria, data gathering would start from the moment of injury and include the following types of information (as examples):

- the injury cause;
- where you were in Victoria;
- whether you were in a car, on a bike or up a ladder;
- the details of your injury (blunt or penetrating, head, spinal, burn, fracture of a limb);
- the hospital you went to, whether you got there by road or air and how long it took;
- all the episodes of care received before and during your hospital stay, when you were discharged and where to; and
- the extent of your long-term physical and mental recovery.[178]

This data is fed to an overarching State Trauma Committee with representation from hospitals, ambulance and retrieval services, the major emergency medicine, nursing and surgical colleges, the TAC and the Department of Health and Human Services (Appendix 6). The Committee uses the data to strategically plan research, policy and modifications designed to optimise system performance. Figure 7 shows the initial governance structure put in place for the VSTS.[179]

Data is also an invaluable insurance against knee-jerk reactions. For example, even in the best trauma systems, patients will die; some injuries are just too great to overcome. Some of these deaths will occur during transport to hospital. The VSTS changed the way patients were transported – in some cases, by sending them to a major trauma service that is further away from the nearest hospital

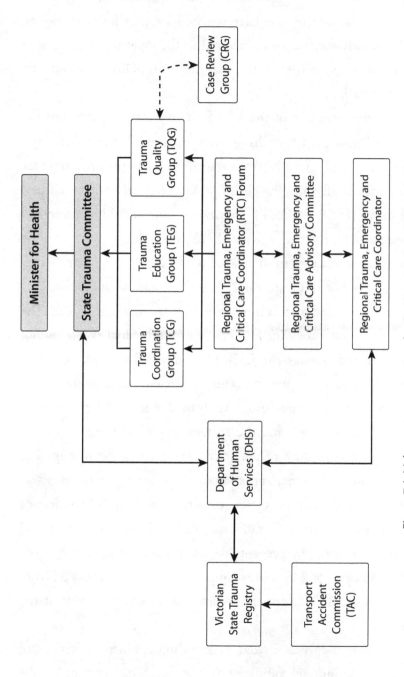

Figure 7: Initial governance structure for the Victorian State Trauma System.

Note the State Trauma Committee reports directly to the Health Minister, and receives input about performance from several different sources, including the registry and case reviews.

From Trauma towards 2014 report (2009)[159]

(the 'volume-outcome' argument). If a patient dies on the way to The Alfred, when he or she may have reached another hospital sooner, it would be easy for people to intuit that the system is failing, and easier still to imagine the adverse publicity and political fallout that this could entail.

Early in the evolution of the VSTS, such isolated events had the potential to "blow the whole thing out of the water." (Peter Cameron, December 2 2016)[177] Deaths from trauma are a terrible outcome for everyone – family, friends, the health professionals who tried their best – an outcome that the CCRTF showed can and should be prevented wherever possible. But the registry places each individual death in the context of the whole system. It enables the Committee to identify that yes, one person died in transit over here; but here is data on the several other lives saved by reaching definitive trauma care earlier. The importance of data providing this context to individual events cannot be overestimated. Just as the CCRTF compelled decisive action to create the VSTS, the registry prevented adverse reaction against it.

The early data was encouraging. Analysis of over 2700 cases between 2001 and 2003 showed that the system was performing largely as designed, with over 80% of major trauma cases being managed at the major trauma services, and a small reduction in death rates was observed.[180] As the numbers grew over the years, so did confidence that the reduction in death rates was real and not just a statistical aberration.[181] Potentially preventable death rates also fell from 36% (based on analysis of 245 deaths immediately prior to the VSTS) to 28% (analysis of 193 deaths immediately after establishment of the VSTS).[182]

This positive data was crucial to guarding against any claims of early system failure by validated the overarching concept of the

VSTS itself – a system reform that was not without controversy due to its unprecedented scope.

Data to optimise system performance

The use of feedback to enhance performance is well established in health systems – in fact, it is one of the most researched strategies to optimise healthcare quality. 'Audit and feedback,' defined as "a summary of clinical performance of health care over a specified period of time"[183] – has been the focus of approximately 140 randomised controlled trials. Collectively, these trials show that providing audit and feedback works to improve healthcare, with effects generally small but consistent across trials, and similar in magnitude to other strategies, for example computerised reminders.[183,184]

The registry enables large-scale audit and feedback, with an annual report presenting a detailed breakdown of the number and types of major trauma cases across Victoria, the key indicators of pre-hospital and hospital performance against evidence-based standards, and the aggregate outcomes for all Victorians involved in major trauma, including long-term recovery for those in the registry for several years. Architects of the registry need only to point to the outcome data to demonstrate the viability of audit and feedback on this scale.

Data had already been used to justify the creation of the VSTS and validate that the new system reduced deaths. But, important as these were, the data could do more than this. Data didn't just show deaths being reduced – it showed where the system and its component parts could be improved to further enhance the care delivered. Data showed how an individual hospital performed against guidelines for care and state-wide benchmarks. Like an aeroplane cockpit, data could highlight system function and identify issues that need to be addressed – response times in a geographical area; a need for more infrastructure; a process that wasn't working as it should; a human resource need that hadn't been fully identified. In doing so, data drew clinicians away from anecdote and beliefs and towards 'flying the plane'. In doing so, it mobilised them around their ultimate goal – to give patients the best possible care that they can.

Of course, every case is different: the circumstances of each accident are unique, patients vary in their age and may or may not carry other health conditions influencing the outcome of care. But over time, hard data that is continuously increasing in volume "moulds people to the mean" (Peter Cameron, December 2 2016).[177] And just like the feedback that we all receive on a daily basis, negative feedback can be confronting, but it is also empowering:

> I know it's mundane; it's not sexy; we all want to be down
> there treating the blood and guts in the emergency room,
> but the actual validation of the registry data is one of the key
> driving points . . . one decision or change based on actual
> data is priceless. And I think that's really the crux of where
> we're heading: we need to have our data and use it so that
> we can make changes for the better (Christine Allsopp,
> New South Wales Trauma System Monitoring Manager,
> November 2011)[185]

As the registry consolidated and grew, so too did the insights. A major review of the VSTS published in 2009 resulted in an overhaul of the patient retrieval system and also recommended greater communication to referring hospitals regarding patient outcomes; and review and updating of guidelines, governance arrangements, data collection and overall system issues and resources.[159]

But perhaps the most critical function of the registry has been its effect on long-term trauma management. Initially, patients in the registry were followed up for six months. Now it is two years. Victoria today houses the world's richest database on recovery, independence and function following trauma. This has forced a widening of the focus on trauma care from 'life versus death' to later stages of trauma care such as long-term rehabilitation.

The registry can also reflect other changes over time. Major trauma is not just road accidents – it is any event resulting in severe injury. The population is aging and this means comparatively more major trauma from falls by the elderly compared to car accidents. Elderly patients have more pre-existing health conditions, managed by a variety of medications. This makes them a different, more complex population than the prototypical young male speeding driver. Imaging technologies have also advanced considerably since inception of the VSTS – meaning that more injuries are being identified in older, sicker people. The registry can measure how the system performs given these demographic and clinical changes, and identify where modifications are needed as these new injury patterns across the Victorian population emerge.[177]

> . . . if data is collected for the system, interpreted and enacted, it becomes a very powerful tool and that's what we've been able to engineer in Victoria." (Peter Cameron, November 2011)[186]

Data about system effectiveness

The headlines tell a compelling story of success and describe a trauma system that is rightly the envy of the world.

Peter Cameron: Counting and being accountable

By Melissa Merino

It's hard to believe Professor Peter Cameron when he says he's "not really a data freak." This after all is the man who played a large part in the establishment of the Victorian State Trauma Registry – a database recording details of injuries sustained from virtually every major trauma in the state.

But the eminent trauma physician and academic director of The Alfred Emergency and Trauma Centre does admit he has a considerable appreciation for the insights this particular set of numbers reveals.

"It's a beautiful thing," says Cameron, who is chief investigator on the registry he helped design and implement, that at once underpins, monitors and guides the Victorian State Trauma System (VSTS). "I've certainly become more data-conscious than when I started emergency medicine."

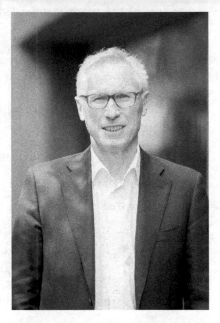

Peter Cameron, October 2017
Image supplied by Kirsten Marks, taken by Gerard Hynes from Hynesite Photography

Established alongside the VSTS, the registry records details not only of road accidents, but 99 per cent of all trauma events, tracking the journey of victims from the time of their accident, all through their treatment and beyond, providing unparalleled insights into the system – and enabling optimal patient outcomes.

Simply, Victoria's much-lauded trauma system wouldn't work without it, Cameron says. "You can't manage the system without the data," he says. "Because without the data you don't know what you're doing."

The particular beauty Cameron most admires about data is that it is irrefutable; objectively illustrating whether the system is working effectively on a macro and micro level – both as a whole as well as the elements within it.

Without data you only have opinions and those opinions can be driven by political or personal agendas, he says. But with data underlying it, the system can be established effectively. "It's really the foundation of the whole system – that it is based on fact rather than someone's opinion," he says. "And early-on it confirmed the system was working."

But Cameron's appreciation for data in fact blossomed well before the existence of the VSTS. Under the guidance of mentor and former Director of the Emergency and Trauma Centre at The Alfred Hospital, Linus Dziukas, and head of Monash University's Department of Epidemiology and Preventive Medicine, John McNeil, Cameron's doctoral thesis combined and analysed data from the early 1990s, for the first time, from all trauma patients across all hospitals in Victoria, to get a handle of the big picture.

Little did he know at the time, but this research, "the first attempt at having a regional dataset of major trauma anywhere in the world of that magnitude", would be used a few years later as the epidemiological evidence on trauma patients by the Robert Doyle chaired taskforce that produced the blueprint for the VSTS itself.

The role that data played in shaping the taskforce's Review of the Trauma and Emergency Services (RoTES) report that built the case for the VSTS cannot be underestimated, Cameron says. And he should know. By then, in the late 1990s, as the Director of the Emergency Department at the Royal Melbourne Hospital, he was himself a Taskforce member.

"When you have a massive change like that, the thing that makes people say 'Yes' or 'No' is whether you know what you are talking about and whether it's based on data," he says. "And we were actually in a position to tell people – 'Well this is what the data says and this is how it would work,' because we knew."

The data not only unequivocally supported the need for a coordinated trauma system, but also informed the design of the system, for instance, in the number and location of specialist trauma centres, and where they should be.

"It was one of the best political-come-health related taskforces that I've been involved with, because it was totally about: 'What is the evidence? What is the data? What do we need?'" Cameron says.

Importantly the blueprint also included within it a mechanism for data to play a continuing role – through a monitoring system tracking trauma cases for the new VSTS – a monitoring system that would become the Victorian State Trauma Registry.

"I knew because of the work I'd been doing – how important the data was – that it was fundamental to the system working," he says. "You can't manage the system without it."

Cameron was part of the tender to develop the registry, with Professor McNeil. And to this day, operating with funding from the TAC through the Victorian Department of Human Services, it reports to the State Trauma

Committee, recording information on every major trauma patient in the state (unless a patient opts out) from the time of their incident to several years after hospital discharge.

The data, he says, has become just as important as the system it underpins. Not simply a passive recording of results, it provides insight into whether the system is working, from hospitals' compliance with guidelines to the effectiveness of clinical practice. And in world-first methodology, tracking patients for two years, it is also providing invaluable information about longer-term outcomes.

"We have demonstrated that not only are we saving lives – we are improving functional outcomes (in surviving patients). And if functional outcomes improve commensurate with the mortality improvements that's a wonderful thing," Cameron says. "And we can show with real evidence this impact we've had over the time of the development of the system because we have the data."

However, any examination of the success of the VSTS in its first decade must account for what had been achieved prior to its introduction, as well as other road safety initiatives during the decade after its inception. In research, a decade is an eternity. Change observed over a long period of time creates an argument about 'causation or association.' A rooster doesn't cause the sun to rise, it just happens to crow around the same time. How can we truly know of the effect of the VSTS?

The Victorian road toll in 1969 was 1034 in a population of 3.4 million – a rate of 30 per 100,000. In 1999, 384 Victorians died on the road in a population of 4.7 million – or 8 per 100,000. This reduction of two-thirds of the rate is a broad reflection of the combined success of the initiatives of the preceding three decades, as illustrated in Figure 8.

Of course, the road safety world didn't stand still in the decade after the introduction of the VSTS. Between December 2000 and

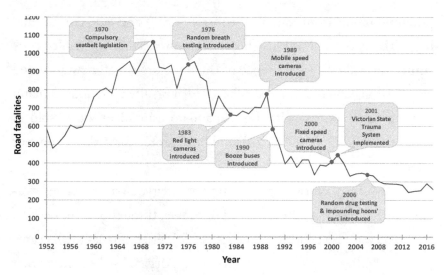

Figure 8: Road trauma deaths in Victoria, Australia (1952–2017) &
associated legislative interventions
Figure by Russell Gruen, data from Transport Accident Commission

July 2002, a major package of measures focused on speed was implemented including the expansion of use and refinements of speed
cameras, the introduction of a 50 km/h general urban speed limit
(40km/h in school and shopping zones) and a restructuring of fines.
Collectively, these were estimated to be responsible for a reduction of
just over eight fatal crashes per month.[80] Approximately $240 mil-
lion was spent improving roads in accident 'blackspot' areas between
2000 and 2004. In 2006, Victoria achieved another legislative world
first – random drug testing and impounding of dangerously driven
(hoon's) cars.[56]

A major 2004 report in vehicle safety estimated that substantial
(20–40%) reductions in serious road trauma would result from adoption of safer car technologies.[187] This spawned an innovative TAC
campaign, 'how safe is your car', which highlighted the life-saving

potential of electronic stability control (ESC) and side curtain air-bags. The associated website (howsafeisyourcar.com.au) enabled consumers to evaluate the presence of these features in all new and used cars.[56] In an echo of *Declare war on 1034*, it resulted in public demand driving public policy, with ESC mandatory in all new cars sold in Australia from December 2010, and head protecting airbags one year later.[100]

A 10-year Victorian road safety strategy, 'Arrive Alive,' was launched in February 2008.[70] And of course, throughout this decade, the TAC was also continuing its successful series of mass media campaigns highlighting key road safety issues, driven by detailed market research.

Teasing out the specific effect of the VSTS and its registry-driven improvements in care from these myriad other initiatives – like identifying the key ingredient of successful parenting in the first decade of a child's life – is of course, impossible. Many of those with a focus on outcomes rather than process, including road trauma survivors, probably don't care and would say 'it's academic.' It's true, the registry is an academic project, but there are many with vested interests in this question, especially the TAC and the Victorian Government. Even though there is no true 'control' group with which to compare, it is this data that will provide the evidence as to whether the VSTS is a major driver of the incredible reduction in risk of death witnessed in Victoria during 2000–2010.

First and foremost is, of course, the registry data. Data from the early years of introduction of the VSTS – even before all hospitals were contributing their records – demonstrated two key facts. First, the system was operating as intended: over 80% of major trauma patients were being transported to the major trauma services.[180]

Second, reductions in system deficiencies were recorded, along with reductions in preventable deaths.[182] In the ensuing years, data has shown a consistent pattern of improvements in trauma processes at the same time as improvements in trauma outcomes. For example, the creation of the Adult Retrieval Service, which centralised the coordination of major trauma patient transfers from accident scene to hospitals, led to a measurable impact on risk of death.[188]

All of these findings are generated from within Victoria, and therefore subject to 'causation versus association' arguments. However, widening of the lens beyond Victoria further supports the differential effect of an organised trauma system. Data from other states that introduced similar state-wide approaches to trauma care, such as South Australia, also demonstrated reductions in risk of death.[189] Comparison to similar first-world countries without an organised trauma system, such as England and Wales at the time the comparison was made, showed superior outcomes from major trauma in Victoria.[164]

Finally, we return to the early studies justifying the introduction of the VSTS. An examination of over 439,000 car accident deaths in the United States from 1979–1995 found that death rates in states with organised trauma systems were 11.6 per 100,000, compared to 15.4 per 100,000 in those without organised systems. Furthermore, this analysis found that the influence of seat belt, license revocation and alterations in speed limits, although associated with alterations in mortality (including a rise where speed limits were raised), did not substantially alter the estimates of how effective the trauma systems were.[190]

Many interstate and overseas jurisdictions without trauma systems have shared the benefits of advances in car safety and have a broadly comparable road law enforcement framework. For this reason, the data on the effect of organised trauma care is compelling such juris-dictions to implement trauma systems, in many cases using Victoria as their template, based on the stunning outcomes achieved in the first decade since implementation of the VSTS.[166] This, combined with the above studies, shows that the VSTS can rightly claim to have been a major – if not the major – contributor to halving the risk of death on Victoria's roads in just one decade; an impact almost unheard of in other areas of medicine.

Data is the glue that binds the creation of the VSTS with measure-ment of its impact. This in turn underpins its viability and enables the system to identify and respond to signals to refine and improve over time. In an era where registries and 'big data' are now not just buzzwords but foundational elements of large healthcare quality improvement efforts, the data from the VSTS, especially regarding long-term outcomes of severe trauma, is internationally significant. The genius of the VSTS lies not just in the VSTS itself, but in the building into that system of a world-first registry capturing detailed information on major trauma outcomes.

This registry is the system-within-a-system that generates the headlines, reduces the power of anecdote, reassures governments and funders, and drives continuous quality improvement. It is the system that tells the ending of the incredible story of the VSTS, which began three decades before its inception. And the beginning of new chapters responding to the quantum shifts that the next wave of technology will bring to motorised transport.

Chapter 6

SURVIVAL

Eventually I think we saw the 'joys'
of change management sit behind us,
and the pleasure of working in a really mature,
high-functioning system become our
day-to-day reality.

(Marcus Kennedy, November 2011)[151]

Since 1996 the Alfred Trauma Service has provided emergency medical support to the Australian Formula One Grand Prix at nearby Albert Park in Melbourne. For four days in March, the event boasts high performance in almost everything – the drivers, the pit crews, the event logistics, the car technologies, and the fashion. The chequered flag waves for the driver who, on the day, has the skills, the team and the equipment that perform the best overall.

And so it is with trauma care. In Chapter 5 we reported the achievements of the VSTS, how thousands of lives have now been saved by an integrated system of care in which individuals and teams perform at a high level. In the preceding chapters we described how this came to be, through building public awareness, creating financial capacity, aligning political, professional and public interests, and using preventable mortality as a spark to to create a better system. In this chapter we look at what has happened since, at what keeps the system going and how it has adapted to a changing world and its own success.

High performance trauma care

Everyone admires high-performance. Performance is something we can measure, and performing well makes us feel good about ourselves and about the things we do. From ballet to racing cars, and from school exams to marathons, high-performance makes us think about what perfection might be like, what it would be like if we didn't make mistakes, and what it is to push the limits of human achievement. It makes us think about systems in which each component does exactly what it is supposed to do, and works seamlessly with other parts that are doing the same. Simply put, high performance is about being the best we can be; doing the best we can do.

For the Victorian paramedics, nurses, doctors and others involved in the immediate care of severely injured patients, high-performance is self-motivating. They recognise the privilege of working in a system that consistently produces exceptional actions that make a real differ-ence to patients' lives. For some it is a calling, for others just a job, but for all it involves nights and weekends, uncertain and out-of-control scenarios, lives hanging in the balance, distraught families, time crit-ical decisions, and some of the sickest patients imaginable. They are action-oriented professionals drawn to the challenges in trauma care, and through their world-class training and experience, most achieve a very high level of individual performance.

Yet they also know that it is usually the team's performance that matters more than the individual's. In sport a high performing team is the one which scores the highest. In logistics a high performing team consistently delivers on time. Similarly, high performing trauma teams are those that save the most lives and consistently achieve good outcomes. For ambulance and hospital trauma clinicians in particular, it is obvious that every life saved has tangible contributions from many people and different specialties.

It is usually apparent to team members when teamwork is good and when it isn't. Many studies have examined the efficiency of trauma teams using human factors approaches and analysis of staff movement. The Alfred Trauma Service has video-recorded thousands of patient resuscitations to identify opportunities for improvement, and have shown that, in the complex and potentially chaotic initial assessment and management of severely injured patients, there is a clear association between individual and team performance, and patient outcomes.[175]

Individual and team performances are critical but, as we've shown in this book, they are, alone, insufficient: high-performance trauma care also requires a system capable of organising and coordinating such care. This is where analogies with sport, logistics and even other medical specialties are less relevant.

High-performing trauma systems

In Formula One there is one common racetrack, every car has four wheels and a similar shape, and they all start at the same time. In trauma care every patient is different. Young and old, short and tall, skinny and obese, they bring myriad body shapes and pre-existing health problems. Their mechanisms of injury have all been different, and they have injuries in different patterns and different severity.

In Victoria motor vehicle crashes and falls predominate, with blunt force leading to many possible organ system injuries, brain injury and spinal cord injuries. In places where gun violence is more common, victims present with isolated penetrating injuries. All of these factors affect the likelihood of survival and recovery, regardless of the quality of the trauma care each patient receives.

Furthermore, within any jurisdiction, even if patients and their injury patterns were identical, the playing field is not level. An injury at the Australian Grand Prix has a waiting medical crew and a journey of 500 metres to a designated Major Trauma Centre, whereas the driver who comes off the road in the rural Victorian highlands may not be discovered for hours, time during which the prospects of survival dwindle as the blood seeps uncontrolled from his or her circulation.

A truly high-performing trauma system responds well in all injury situations, irrespective of precise geographic location, pre-existing health status, type and severity of injuries, and number of casualties. A critical part of the system is the capability to rapidly determine each patient's needs and provide the necessary care. Life saving measures first, and subsequent care that doesn't overlook anything. Every country faces challenges in creating such systems. This is, in part, because health care systems are built to deal best with well-defined conditions with established management guidelines, or multiple chronic conditions that don't demand immediate treatment. In trauma care, the system must cope rapidly with everything from a simple fracture to an unconscious patient with multiple hidden but life-threatening internal injuries. A different paradigm is needed.

In 2013 the World Health Organization's Global Alliance for Care of the Injured defined the three goals of essential trauma care that define this paradigm: 1. Life-saving care at the scene; 2. Timely treatment of injuries, and 3. Restoration of function and independence.

The first goal incorporates the fundamentals of response and resuscitation – the 'ABC' of first aid, emphasising that airway obstruction, failure of ventilation and active bleeding are treatable and underpin many preventable deaths. As a trauma system goal, it invites consideration of who potential responders could be – lay persons, community members with special training, ambulance paramedics, and physicians who travel to the scene. Each system is different – the mainstay of Victoria's pre-hospital system are highly-trained ambulance paramedics with advanced airway and haemorrhage control skills.

The second goal – timely treatment of injuries – underlines the importance of prioritisation, of sometimes making treatment decisions such as going to the operating theatre without waiting to know precise diagnoses if it seems that major bleeding is present. It also emphasises the need to minimise unnecessary delays to optimal treatment – for example by transport to a facility that is unable to properly manage the patient – and minimise the risk of missing injuries. An undiagnosed wrist fracture, for example, may cause a patient chronic pain years after surviving her multiple life-threatening injuries.

The Victorian system invested in predetermined pre-hospital triage and transport protocols based on individual patients' needs, mobilising whatever resources were required: helicopter ambulances, road car, even fixed wing aircraft, to respond most appropriately. Once the patient reaches hospital the reception and resuscitation is also highly protocolised, with advanced notification of arrival, designated response teams, standard procedures, checklists, and repeated examinations all promoting timeliness of treatment and minimising delayed diagnoses and missed injuries.

The third goal – restoration of function and independence – highlights that, for seriously injured patients, the challenges don't end at discharge from hospital. Instead many face a long road to rebuild their lives, and many will have permanent physical or mental impairment. The latest annual data from the Victorian State Trauma System Outcomes Registry indicates that since 2010, only 30% of adults and 40% of children have made a good recovery from major trauma (defined as returning to their pre-injury level of function with few or no residual problems).[191]

Previously underappreciated, we have better understanding of the long-term burden because the Registry collects information from patients after they've left hospital, and during their journey over months and years to regain function and independence, as seen in Table 1. This information opens up new opportunities to improve long-term care and support.

Table 1: Medium to long-term outcomes of survivors of major trauma in Victoria based on data collected on over 2,000 cases from 2006–2010.[160]

Outcome	Time since injury		
	6 months (%)	12 months (%)	24 months (%)
Complete functional recovery	18.1	22.3	27.9
Return to work	61.6	68.6	72.2
Moderate to severe pain	21.0	20.0	20.0
Moderate to severe disability – physical health (PCS-12)	45.3	40.5	37.4
Moderate to severe disability – mental health (MCS-12)	22.2	23.0	20.4

Belinda Gabbe: Lives worth living

By Bianca Nogrady

As a physiotherapist, Professor Belinda Gabbe knows the importance of long-term follow-up. But every once in a while, a patient comes along and illustrates that need with crystal clarity.

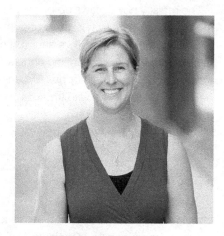

Belinda Gabbe, February 2018
Image supplied by Kirsten Marks,
taken by Gerard Hynes from
Hynesite Photography

This time, it was a patient who had experienced a major traumatic injury. They had been discharged from hospital, but were still suffering serious pain. Desperate for help, but not sure where to turn, they had even rung the number for the ethics body listed among information sent to patients on the Victorian State Trauma Registry.

The ethics contact reached out to Gabbe, who passed on the telephone number for the care coordinator at the hospital where the patient had originally been treated. "Within 15 minutes, I got a text message back from that care coordinator saying 'I've spoken to the patient, we already have a plan in place, everything is looking good'," she recalls.

This experience highlights the importance of Gabbe's research at the Victorian State Trauma Registry. As an Australian Research Centre Future Fellow and head of the Pre-Hospital, Emergency and Trauma Research Unit at Monash University, she is investigating the care and long-term outcomes for people who have been hospitalised with major traumatic injury.

The hope is that this research will not only lead to a better understanding of life after traumatic injury, but lay an evidence-based foundation for better care and follow-up systems to ensure that patient care continues for as long as it is needed.

Major trauma is the very definition of an acute medical situation; it's fast, intense and severe. In such a setting, short-term survival is the name of the game, so the outcomes measured have tended to be short-term ones; if survivors could walk, talk and feed themselves when they were discharged from hospital, that was a win. But that wasn't enough for Gabbe.

"If I'd survived serious injury I'd want to return to work and return to social and leisure activities, and get my life back on track," she says. "But unless we measured that, we would never know whether we were really having good outcomes for our patients and whether they were living a life that they were happy with."

The registry now follows up by telephone with all trauma patients at six months, one year and two years after they leave hospital, and in a smaller group of patients for up to five years after discharge.

The work is already changing understanding of the long-term impact of major trauma, which until recently has focused largely only on long-term disability in people who were living with traumatic brain or spinal cord injury, as opposed to other forms of major trauma.

"What we've discovered is that the recovery trajectories for patients are actually really long, complex processes, and we now understand that people don't just get better or plateau – they can actually get worse over time as well," Gabbe says.

In reality, major trauma behaves more like a chronic disease than an acute condition, and Gabbe says that needs to be reflected in the structure of medical services for major trauma patients. While the Victorian State Trauma System is world-class, the Australian health system isn't always the easiest to navigate, and people can slip through the cracks – like the patient with trauma-related persistent pain.

"From the point of view of the outcomes of patients, I'd really like to see that we have established single points of contact or care coordinators for all of the major trauma patients around the state," Gabbe says.

In the meantime, the registry – while technically being a population-based monitoring tool for the trauma system – has also found itself occasionally playing the role of de facto care coordinator.

"If you're on a call to a patient and they really are having trouble, ethically and morally you can't leave that patient," she says. So resource packages and algorithms have been developed for the registry, to guide telephone interviewers through what to do if patients are distressed and need help.

It's not about providing clinical care, but instead giving people advice on where to find help, how to contact clinical services and, in some cases, contacting those services on the patient's behalf.

The registry is also earning international attention, particularly from the United Kingdom and the United States, which are looking to include long-term outcomes in their national trauma databases.

But for Gabbe, the most rewarding aspect of the work is being able to give people a voice when their recovery might not be going so well, and to help that voice be heard at all levels.

"We're starting to see a real move towards improving the outcomes for patients through better care coordination and accessibility to services," Gabbe says. "Having that direct line into working with policy makers and key stakeholders, like the Department of Health and Human Services and the Transport Accident Commission, has been fantastic."

In combination, the data that showed improved survival and reduction in preventable deaths, and the previously unrecognised long-term burden of injury, was to catalyse another seismic shift in policy. And again, it was the TAC that drove it.

Changing priorities

The implementation of the VSTS in 2001 was a landmark event in Victoria. But it wasn't the end of the story. The system has not stood still.

Established in response to an epidemic of road trauma, the VSTS was predicated especially on the public, professional and political revulsion at the news that injured Victorians were dying unnecessarily. Awareness of preventable deaths led to significant investment in ambulance and hospital emergency departments. Considerable gains in the quality and consistency of trauma patient reception and resuscitation were achieved. Within a decade the likelihood of a patient dying from his injuries had been halved, an extraordinary health outcomes achievement on par with penicillin for sepsis and anti-retroviral drugs for HIV. While the CCRTF has not been formally reconvened, every trauma death in Victoria is still audited, and almost all are deemed non-preventable. The majority of trauma fatalities have suffered non-survivable brain injuries. Once injury has occurred, preventable and potentially avoidable deaths are now very uncommon.

This achievement was noted and celebrated by clinical groups and governors of the system. But inevitably the near elimination of preventable deaths led to a strong perception that further investment in the early trauma response may not continue to reap benefits. At the same time, the Victorian State Trauma Outcomes Registry (VSTORM) was bringing forward post-hospital data about the ongoing pain and disability faced by severely injured patients, and their difficulties with returning to work and regaining independence.

The focus of policy-makers' and payers' attention shifted, and the TAC was a catalyst. Through the Victorian Trauma Foundation (VTF), the TAC had contributed to trauma research with an emphasis on early care. As the cost burden of TAC clients with brain or spinal cord injury became apparent – lifetime estimates of $5 million and $10 million per case, respectively[192] – the VTF was replaced in 2005 with the Victorian Neurotrauma Initiative (VNI), to which the TAC contributed $60 million for brain and spinal cord injury research up until 2010. Most of this was directed towards understanding and improving long-term care.

In 2010 the TAC formalised a new research institute, the Institute for Safety, Compensation and Recovery Research (ISCRR), launched in 2011,[193] and also launched its Recovery and Independence divisions to be able to better provide for its clients by tailoring services to an appropriate and realistic level of possible recovery for each patient. The latter included the introduction of a client-centred Independence Plan and greater engagement of TAC case managers with health and lifetime care providers.[194]

New public and private providers emerged, and the State Trauma Committee's remit came to include, to some degree at least, the performance and efficiency of long-term care providers. By 2015, rehabilitation and long-term care services had become an integral part of the Victorian State Trauma System, and the majority of research and development funding had moved from prehospital and emergency care to the long-term care of patients, where greatest efficiency gains for Government were thought to lie. What funding did get allocated to improve trauma reception and resuscitation was directed mostly to educational resources for rural clinicians. The system had come of age.

Just as in 1999–2001, bringing about such changes was helped by patient stories. For example the 2015–2016 VSTORM Report told the story of Gino's car crash, the prehospital and hospital-based care he received for his head, chest and abdominal injuries, his post-hospital recovery in a rehabilitation facility, and his eventual return to work with minimal residual disability.[191] Similarly, dedicated doctors, nurses and allied health personnel were just as much part of the story. But unlike the development of the VSTS in the first place, the shift in emphasis from early care to long term care wasn't led by concerned clinicians or an outraged public. This was a quieter revolution, informed by data, driven by the TAC as a funder, and led by policy-makers and economic imperatives. It was no less effective, though – the system continues to thrive, the road toll continues to decline, and the quality of survival will likely continue to improve.

A sustainable and adapting system

Put together, the evolution of the VSTS over the past two decades is best understood as a complex adaptive system involving the community, health care services, injured patients, and the funders and policy-makers. The nature of each element and the interactions

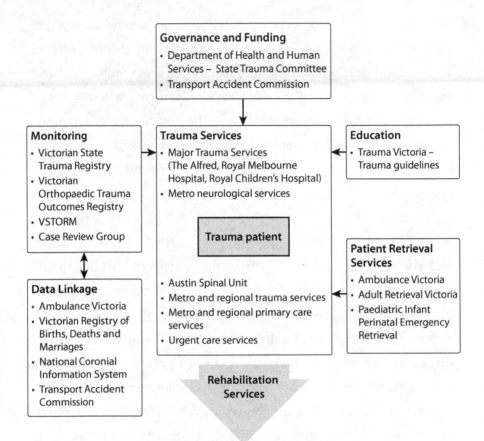

Figure 9: The current structure of the Victorian State Trauma System
Source: Victorian State Trauma Outcome Registry and Monitoring Group (2017)[191]

between them have had an important bearing on the relevance, performance and sustainability of the system (Figure 9).

A complex adaptive systems model developed specially to guide the sustainability of health programs (Figure 10) is helpful in understanding what happened, and planning for the future. This model requires us to define the actors in the system: those who provide care (trauma care services), the recipients of that care (severely injured people), the drivers that can exert influence over the system

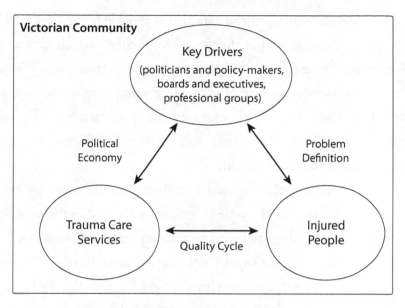

Figure 10: The VSTS as a complex adaptive system
(Adapted from Gruen RL 2008)[195]

(politicians and policymakers in a public systems, boards and executives in private systems, and others such as powerful professional groups), and the broader community (of taxpayers, shareholders, potential patients and myriad interested organisations).

The model also directs our attention to the relationships between entities. Clinicians and patients most often concentrate on how well the care provided meets patients' needs, and how patients' needs change as care is provided. In an individual clinical situation, this can be thought of as how controlling a bleeding artery saves a patient's life, allowing focus on other non-life-threatening injuries. At system level, improved prehospital care and faster transport to hospital enables earlier life-saving surgical control of bleeding, resulting in more patients surviving and needing beds in the ICU where their other injuries will be managed.

The association between the care that is provided, and how well it achieves its goals, as well as the downstream effects which in trauma often create demand for other care, is referred to as the 'quality cycle'. It makes us consider how well the care is meeting the needs of injured patients and how might it be improved. The Victorian State Trauma Registry, and audits of outcomes, such as the CCRTF, are the main repositories of this information.

How this information is used is reflected in the other parts of the model. Trauma services use information about effectiveness and ongoing needs to advocate for more resources into the program. The way they engage with the key drivers, such as Members of Parliament, the Victorian Department of Human Services and the TAC, and how that influences the flow of resources, is 'the political economy' of trauma care.

Of course such stakeholders' decisions depend on their perceptions and priorities for limited resources. This is the 'problem definition' component of the model. Key drivers can also shape public opinion and how others perceive the needs. Adversarial party politics can easily lead to politicisation of issues based on anticipated electoral appeal.

The model is useful for understanding how Victoria's trauma system has successfully invented and reinvented itself. From 1970, thanks to Harry Gordon's campaign in *The Sun*, publication of the road toll, and the TACs very effective mass media campaigns, the Victorian community was increasingly aware that road trauma was a significant problem. *The Sun* and the TAC successfully used public opinion to embolden politicians towards new injury prevention and trauma care legislation. The CCRTF data, its publications and its presentation to Government Ministers added, as a powerful extra dimension, the idea that the healthcare system was failing to the point that people with survivable injuries were dying unnecessarily. And the CCRTF mobilised influential professional groups to demand change.

In the late 1990s the problem was sufficiently defined, the alarm sufficiently loud, a critical financial enabler – the TAC – was in place, and the key drivers were sufficiently aligned and motivated. Major service changes ensued, initiated through the Review of Trauma and Emergency Services (the RoTES Report), and subsequent birth of the new system. John Thwaites, the new Health Minister presented with the decision of whether or not to implement the recommendations of the RoTES Report, summed up the importance of problem definition and the key drivers when he indicated his confidence that "not only were they the right recommendations but there'd also be wide support for them across the health community."

The new system strengthened ambulance and hospital-based services, system governance, and a new registry containing high-quality data about injured patients and their care. The registry showed rapid reduction in road deaths, justifying the decision and emboldening the community to strive for further road toll reductions.

Importantly, the Victorian State Trauma Registry also pioneered the collection and analysis of information about medium and long-term outcomes, and for the first time anywhere a comprehensive picture of the burden of injury was visible. A different set of problems was evident – defined by patients' ongoing pain and suffering, use of health care services, time off work and, in cases of brain, spinal cord or major orthopaedic injuries, dependence on long-term supportive care. Compared to preventable deaths in the healthcare system, these problems were less dramatic and unlikely to raise public outrage, but analyses showed them to have major human and economic costs, for which new, more efficient practices were needed. Furthermore, they would not be solved by additional investment in ambulance and emergency departments. Instead these problems demanded attention to the post-hospital care, rehabilitation, and community-based services. Again the TAC was a major actor, this time making a direct case to Treasury about the cost of long-term care and lost productivity.

More an evolution than a revolution, reprioritisation from acute up-front critical care to long-term supportive and rehabilitative care was devoid of the fanfare of a new system and lives being saved. But it was no less significant, and vitally important for the patients, families and communities that bore the long-term burdens of injuries.

An eye to the future

Not satisfied with a fourfold reduction in road deaths, the TAC launched its Towards Zero campaign in 2016. It is an integrated approach to reducing deaths and harm from road trauma that in some ways comes full circle, refocusing on injury prevention just as the landmark seatbelt and drink driving initiatives of the 1970s and 1980s did. However now there are new approaches to safe roads, safe speeds, safe vehicles and safe people that draw on modern technology and innovation. Road modifications such as flexible barriers, run-off-road preventions, digital speed and red-light cameras, and car safety features such as electronic stability control, auto emergency braking, lane departure warning, seat belt pre-tensioners, airbags, crumple zones, speed assistance systems have become commonplace. And while driverless cars bring both opportunities and challenges in future mobility, the expectations of collision avoidance technologies are tantalising.

The future of trauma care is no less exciting, and likely to be just as significant in its impact. The major trends will include more rapid provision of time-critical care by bringing diagnostics and treatments to the patient at the roadside, failsafe systems that don't allow errors to occur, more accurate monitoring and diagnostics linked to interventions that are self-actuated, advances in therapeutics for protecting, restoring and regenerating injured tissues, better rehabilitation technologies, and improved care coordination. Precision medicine and point-of-care diagnostics will provide future clinicians with a powerful set of tools for patients unlucky enough to be injured.

The goal of zero road deaths is no longer the stuff of fantasy. It shows how far we've come. In 1969 Victoria had one of the highest per capita road tolls in the world. Today we imagine a future where no-one dies on the road. That we believe it's possible, and that it may be just around the corner, is testament to the success of the Victorian State Trauma System, and all who built it.

Viewed through one lens, the VSTS looks like, and is, reproducible. Viewed through another, it is a system that evolved in the minds of a series of brilliant and dedicated individuals and came to fruition through some key events and lucky coincidences. The upgrade of the coroner's office in response to the Chamberlain case. The pre-existing relationship between Frank McDermott and Robert Doyle, that greased the wheels of the ministerial taskforce. The long-standing bipartisanship that enabled the VSTS to be born soon after an unexpected change of Victorian government. There are many quantifiable and tangible ingredients that could be mixed to recreate the trauma system in other parts of the world and, indeed, this is happening with great success. But the confluence of events and people that gave rise to the VSTS is a story that is unique to Victoria, and perhaps the most magical ingredient of them all.

Political jurisdictions that improve the
organization of trauma services
benefit from reduced trauma mortality,
in comparison with similarly resourced
jurisdictions that do not

(World Health Organization, 2004)[196]

EPILOGUE

By Melissa Marino

Back in January 2010 Micaela Henderson, lying unconscious and bleeding in the aftermath of the car crash, was about to become the beneficiary of the multiple processes put in place as part of the decade-old VSTS.

The first was the ambulance helicopter that arrived to transport her to a designated trauma hospital – in this case the Royal Melbourne – to deal with her severe, life-threatening injuries. And the paramedics arrived not a moment too soon. Weeks later, when she woke from an induced coma, she was told she had died four times, twice at the accident scene and twice in the helicopter – her stopped heart revived by the specialist-trained paramedics who had come to her aid.

On landing at the Royal Melbourne Hospital Micaela was transferred straight to the trauma team who had been briefed on her condition. So severe were her injuries, her parents, who had rushed from their suburban Melbourne home, could only identify her by a small tattoo on her wrist.

"Apparently mum described me as tall and beautiful and blonde," Micaela says. "But because I was so messed up and covered in blood they couldn't tell how tall I was or the colour of my hair or anything else."

With a broken back, shoulder, wrist and elbow, and significant lacerations, Micaela was stabilised for monitoring and assessment. Within 24 hours, that monitoring told the trauma team her brain was swelling, so she underwent emergency surgery in which part of her skull was removed. It wouldn't be replaced for 10 months.

"I had no skull until September or October so I had to wear a helmet. Very attractive," she deadpans.

After successful cranioplasty, Micaela was placed into a coma to help her recover from this and her other injuries. The doctors had advised her parents she would need to be sedated for four weeks but their fit and healthy daughter had other ideas. Not even the powerful medication could keep her down.

"I fought my way out of the coma after two weeks – I kept coming to and not responding to the sedative drugs and eventually they said 'Just wake her up'," she says.

As Micaela gained consciousness and her brain began its recovery, an awareness of what had happened to her slowly came into focus. At the end of April, four months after the crash, she remembers her mother telling her she had been in a serious road accident. To this day, it's the earliest memory she has of the entire experience.

Soon after, she understood the doctors saying she may never walk again. "And they also said I might not be able to balance again, I might never again go water skiing and I thought 'Hmmm – you just watch me'," she says.

And so Micaela, who had by then been shifted to the Epworth Hospital, began her rehabilitation process in earnest.

Overseen and funded by the TAC, which offers a lifetime of cover and support for patients injured on Victoria's roads, she spent eight months in hospital learning to talk, eat, walk and think.

True to her word, she was soon walking unassisted (often sneaking out of her bed and down the corridor) and constructing full sentences. Within two summers, she would water ski again.

Twelve months after the accident, she re-enrolled in university, beginning her studies at Charles Sturt University by correspondence from her parents' home where she had moved after being discharged from hospital.

Rather than staying in agricultural science, she switched to a Bachelor of Agricultural Business Management. "I had decided I didn't want to work on a farm without the option of owning the farm," she quips.

To progress that far, her brain had to re-learn how to learn. For example in reaching for a glass of water an undamaged brain would send a signal to 'a to b to c' to get it done, she explains. "Whereas for me, because those pathways got so messed-up, my brain goes from a to b to f to z, y, m . . . oh c – there we go, we reached it'," she says. "So that's why I get so tired because my brain has to go through so many more pathways to get the end result."

These cerebral pathways gradually become more direct every day as Micaela builds her life with her partner on Queensland's Gold Coast where she recently shifted for the warm weather to ease the pain in her bones that still ache from her injuries. "Even in warmer temperatures I will still sleep with a hot water bottle under my back because it's still pretty sore," she says.

It's been years now since the crash, but her recovery continues, as does the TAC's support, helping financially over the years with physiotherapy, sleep therapy and gym membership to keep strengthening the parts of her body that were affected. She even took part in mindfulness research which helped her understand and counter anxiety she experienced after the crash.

"If you are going to injure yourself – do it on the road," says Micaela, for whom the TAC's support has been "fabulous" in helping her regain an independent life.

So independent is she that she doesn't like to tell people about her crash, especially her colleagues at a national bank where, defying all early expectations of her future working capacity, she recently landed a full-time job.

And this reluctance to mention the accident is not because she doesn't want to think about the experience but because she doesn't want it to alter or limit people's expectations of her. She wants to be judged purely on her merits and not for her progress since the crash – no matter how remarkable.

"Since the accident I have lived as though recovering from it is my biggest achievement and that's not how I want to live anymore," she says. "Right now I couldn't be happier and I couldn't be luckier."

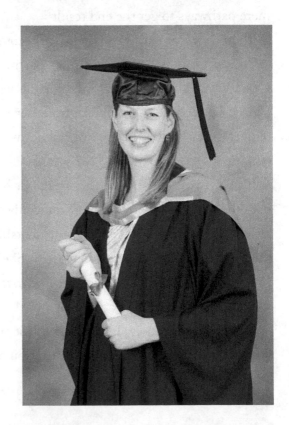

Micaela Henderson graduated with a Bachelor of Agricultural Business Management from Charles Sturt University in December 2016
Image supplied by Micaela Henderson, taken by a professional photographer, Charles Sturt University

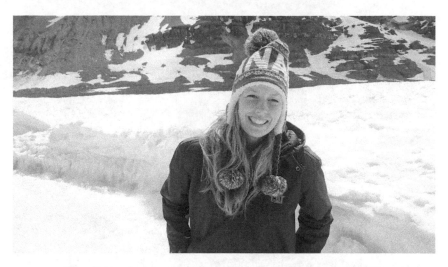

Micaela Henderson on holidays in the United States in May 2015
Image supplied by Micaela Henderson, taken by Tony Henderson

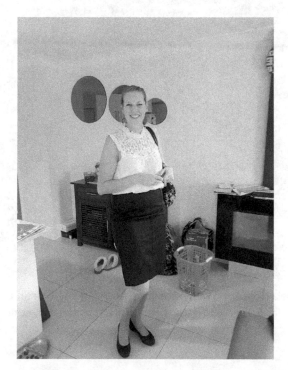

Micaela Henderson on her first day of work in June 2017
Image supplied by Micaela Henderson, taken by Allan Higgins

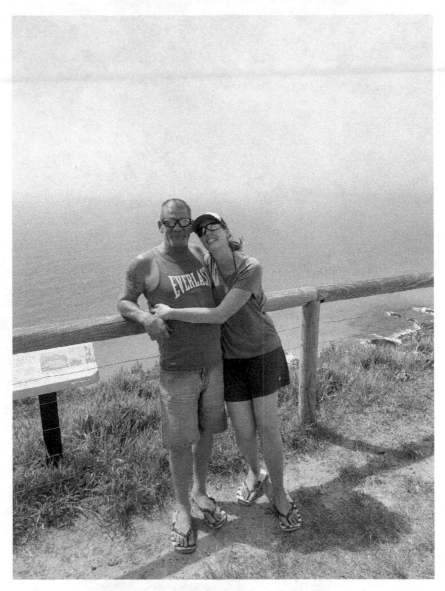

Micaela Henderson with her fiancée Allan Higgins in October 2017
Image supplied by Micaela Henderson, taken by Wendy Keith

APPENDICES

Appendix 1

Victorian Parliamentary Road Safety Committee Inquiries

Sources: Parliament of Victoria,[197] Clark et al. (2005)[4]

Year	Inquiry
1968	Roadworthiness of motor vehicles
1969	Points demerit system
1969	Investigation into the desirability of the compulsory fitting and the compulsory wearing of seat belts
1970	An aspect of the alcohol and drug factor – The desirability of introducing blood alcohol tests at hospitals for certain driver victims of motor vehicle accidents
1970	An aspect of the alcohol and drug factor – The desirability of compulsory breath analysis tests for motor car drivers suspected of having a blood alcohol content in excess of 0.05 per cent
1970	Alcohol and road accidents
1971	Permits for learner drivers
1971	Absolute speed limits, *prima facie* speed limits and speed zones
1972	The Visual Average Speed Computer and Recorder (VASCAR)
1972	Age for driver licensing
1973	Pedestrians and street lighting
1973	An aspect of statistical data for road safety purposes
1974	Aspects of roadworthiness, speedometers, alcohol and road accidents and intersectional management

1975	Alcohol and road safety (research projects involving drinking drivers)
	Fatalities and injuries involving children under 8 who are unrestrained in motor cars
1976	Identification of motor vehicle drivers with blood alcohol levels in excess of .05 per cent
	The involvement of motorcyclists in road accidents
1977	Education, training and assessment of motorcycle learner riders
1978	Impounding of registration plates, penalties for unlicensed driving and some aspects of alcohol and road safety
1979	Mopeds
1980	Safety aspects of the hire and drive omnibus
1981	Restraint of children under 8 in the rear seats of motor cars
	Alcohol prohibition for first year drivers
1983	Freeway speed limits
	Road safety in Victoria (interim report)
1984	Road safety in Victoria (first report)
	Road safety in Victoria (final report)
1986	Child pedestrian & bicycle safety (first report)
	Child pedestrian & bicycle safety 'Safe Roads for Children' (second and final report)
1988	Management of drink-drivers apprehended with high blood alcohol levels 'Alcohol Abuse and Road Safety' (first report)
	Management of drink-drivers apprehended with high blood alcohol levels 'Drink-Driver Education and Treatment' (second and final report)
1990	Vehicle occupant protection
1991	Speed limits in Victoria
1992	Motorcycle safety in Victoria 'Motorcycle Visibility' (first report)
1993	Motorcycle safety in Victoria
1994	Demerit points scheme

1995	Report to the Parliament Upon the Draft Australian Road Rules
	Revision of speed limits in Victoria
	Effects of drugs (other than alcohol) on road safety in Victoria (first report)
1996	Report to the Parliament upon the draft Australian road rules
1995	Effects of drugs (other than alcohol) on road safety in Victoria (final report)
1998	Review of motorcycle safety
1999	Incidence and prevention of pedestrian accidents 'Walking Safely'
2001	Victoria's vehicle roadworthiness system
2002	Rural road safety & infrastructure
2003	Road safety for older road users
2005	Crashes involving roadside objects
	Country road toll
2006	Driver Distraction
	Incidence and Prevention of Pedestrian Accidents
2008	Vehicle safety
	Safety at Level Crossings
2009	Australian Design Rules
2010	Federal-State Road Funding
2012	Motorcycle Safety
2014	Serious Injury

Appendix 2

Members of the Consultative Committee on Road Traffic Fatalities (CCRTF)

Sources: McDermott 2005,[142] 2010[198]

Profession	Affiliation
Pathologists (3)	
Michael Burke	Victorian Institute of Forensic Medicine
Stephen Cordner (Co-Chair)	Victorian Institute of Forensic Medicine
David Ranson	Victorian Institute of Forensic Medicine
General Surgeons (16)	
Chris Atkin	The Alfred Hospital
Wendy Brown	The Alfred Hospital
Paul Cashin	Dandenong Hospital
Narine Efe	The Royal Melbourne Hospital
Richard Gilhome	Dandenong Hospital
Afif Hadj	Maroondah Hospital
Ian Hayes	The Royal Melbourne Hospital
Annette Holianfbrand	The Alfred Hospital
Rodney Judson	The Royal Melbourne Hospital
Thomas Kossman	The Alfred Hospital
Frank McDermott (Co-Chair)	The Alfred Hospital
Cass McInnes	The Alfred Hospital
Julie Miller	The Royal Melbourne Hospital
Peter Ryan	St Vincent's Hospital

Gordon Trinca	Royal Australasian College of Surgeons
Jason Winnett	The Alfred Hospital
Neurosurgeons (5)	
Bhadu Kavar	The Royal Melbourne Hospital
John Laidlaw	The Royal Melbourne Hospital
Patrick Lo	The Royal Children's Hospital
Jeffrey Rosenfeld	The Alfred
Chris Thien	St Vincent's Hospital
Orthopaedic Surgeon (1)	
Garry Grossbard	Box Hill Hospital
Cardiothoracic Surgeons (3)	
Phillip Antippa	The Royal Melbourne Hospital
Bruce Davis	The Alfred Hospital
John Goldblatt	The Royal Melbourne Hospital
Anaesthetists (3)	
Andrew Silvers	The Alfred Hospital
Bill Shearer	Dandenong Hospital
Gerard Stainsby	The Royal Melbourne Hospital
Intensivists (5)	
Warwick Butt	The Royal Children's Hospital
Jamie Cooper	The Alfred Hospital
Grahame Duke	Northern Hospital
Peter Morley	The Royal Melbourne Hospital
John Reeves	Epworth Hospital

Emergency Physicians (5)	
Carolyn Cooper	Austin Repatriation Hospital
Mark Fitzgerald	The Alfred Hospital
Richard Harrod	The Royal Melbourne Hospital
Mark Smith	The Alfred Hospital / Frankston Hospital
Johannes Wenzel	Dandenong Hospital
Ambulance Paramedics (3)	
Murray Barkmeyer	Ambulance Airwing
Greg Cooper	Metropolitan Ambulance Service
Phillip Hogan	Ambulance Airwing
Project Manager (1)	
Ann Tremayne	Consultative Committee on Road Traffic Fatalities

Appendix 3

Members of the Ministerial Taskforce on Trauma and Emergency Services

(Shaded names were also on the Consultative Committee on Road Traffic Fatalities: CCRTF)

Source: Review of Trauma and Emergency Services (1999)[150]

Name	Occupation	Affiliation
Mr Robert Doyle (Chair)	Parliamentary Secretary to the Minister for Health	State Government of Victoria
Dr Frank Archer	Senior Medical Director	Ambulance Service Victoria
Dr Beth Ashwood	Consultant Anaesthetist	Western Hospital
Mr Christopher Atkin	Surgeon in Charge, Trauma Reception	The Alfred Hospital Trauma Service
Professor Ian Brand	Chair	Consultative Council on Emergency and Critical Care Services
Ms Anna Burgess	Manager, Planning and Project Development	North Western Health
Associate Professor Peter Cameron	Director, Emergency Medicine	Royal Melbourne Hospital
Ms Meredith Carter (till July 1998)	Consumer representative	Health Issues Centre
Professor John Catford	Director, Public Health and Development	Department of Human Services
Ms Judith Congalton (till September 1998)	Director of Nursing	St Vincent's Private Hospital
Dr Peter Crossley	Director, Emergency Department	Bendigo Health Care Group
Associate Professor Peter Danne	Director of Trauma Services	Royal Melbourne Hospital

Dr Linus Dziukas	Staff Specialist, Emergency Department	The Alfred
Dr David Eddey	Director, Emergency Department	Geelong Hospital
Mr Elton Edwards	Consultant Orthopaedic Surgeon	The Alfred
Dr Joe Epstein	Director, Emergency Medicine / Coordinator, Emergency and Critical Care Services	North Western Health
Professor Andrew Kaye	Professor of Surgery / Director of Neurosurgery	University of Melbourne / Royal Melbourne Hospital
Dr Marcus Kennedy	Staff Specialist, Emergency Department	Inner and Eastern Health Care Network
Dr Richard King	Director of General Medicine & Emergency Medicine	Southern Health Care Network
Honorary Associate Professor Frank McDermott		Consultative Committee on Road Traffic Fatalities
Dr Campbell Miller	Assistant Director, Acute Health	Department of Human Services (from March 1998)
Dr Peter Morley	Consultant Intensivist and Anaesthetist	Royal Melbourne Hospital
Dr Anna Peeters	Consumer Representative	Health Issues Centre (from July 1998)
Dr Mark Robinson	General Medical Practitioner	Mount Beauty Medical Centre
Associate Professor Jeffrey Rosenfeld	Director of Neurosurgery / Deputy Director of Neurosurgery	Royal Children's Hospital / Royal Melbourne Hospital
Professor Frank Shann	Director, Intensive Care Unit	Royal Children's Hospital

Dr Philip Street	Geriatrician	
Mr Denis Swift	Manager, Health Policy	Transport Accident Commission
Ms Elizabeth Virtue	Nurse Manager, Emergency Department	Western Hospital
Associate Professor Jeff Wassertheil	Director, Emergency Department / Medical Director	Mornington Peninsula Hospital / Ambulance Service Victoria
Associate Professor Bruce Waxman	Director of Academic Surgical Unit	Monash University – Dandenong Hospital
Dr Heather Wellington	Assistant Director, Acute Health	Department of Human Services (till March 1998)
Dr Simon Young	Director, Emergency Services	Royal Children's Hospital
Mr Andrejs Zamurs	Director of Disability Services and Rural Health	Department of Human Services

Appendix 4

Groups within the Ministerial Taskforce on Trauma and Emergency Services

Source: Review of Trauma and Emergency Services (1999)[150]

- Working Party on Emergency and Trauma Services (16 members)
- Retrieval Subgroup (19 members)
- Neurosurgical Subgroup (3 members)
- Education Subgroup (3 members)
- System Monitoring Subgroup (7 members)
- Role Deliniation Subgroup (5 members)
- Paediatric Subgroup (3 members)
- Ambulance Communication Subgroup (6 members)
- Secretariat to Ministerial Review of Trauma and Emergency Services (6 members)

Appendix 5

Other groups and individuals involved in producing the Review of Trauma and Emergency Services (RoTES) report

Source: Review of Trauma and Emergency Services (1999)[150]

- Consultative Committees on Emergency and Critical Care Services and Rural Workforce Agency Victoria
- Specialists who assisted with drafting the specialist trauma transfer guidelines: Mr Rodney Judson, Professor Frank Shann, Dr Simon Young, Associate Professor Jeffrey Rosenfeld, Dr Douglas Brown, Dr Jamie Cooper, Dr Ian Millar, Professor Andrew Kaye, Mr John Laidlaw, Dr Christine Bessell, Mr Elton Edwards and Dr Jenny Dowd.
- Professor Donald Trunkey, Oregon Health Sciences University, Oregon, USA
- Monash University Accident Research Centre
- Ms Ann Tremayne, Consultative Council on Road Traffic Fatalities
- Linda Smart and Dr Ron Manning from NSW Health Department, Dr Tony Burrell, Mike Willis, Dr Andrew Berry, Ian Badham, Trish McDougall and Mr Jim McGrath
- Managers and staff of the following branches of the Department of Human Services: Quality Branch, Acute Health; Purchasing and Financial Policy Branch, Acute Health; Corporate Strategy; Public Health and Development; Communications Unit, Portfolio Services
- Metropolitan Ambulance Service
- Visual Communication Services, The Alfred
- Transport Accident Commission

Appendix 6

The Victorian State Trauma Committee

Source: Victorian Government Department of Health (2013)[179]

Ministerial oversight of the VSTS is facilitated through the State Trauma Committee. The committee provides advice on policy development, system performance and quality management strategies, to support:

- Clear and consistent system response to trauma management
- Definitive care for all patients at an appropriate health service
- Role delineation of health services, including the three major trauma services as centres of excellence
- Coordination and timely transfer of patients
- Education and training in the statewide system organisation and management of trauma response
- System performance monitoring initiatives, including thematic analysis of the Victorian State Trauma System using the Victorian State Trauma Registry to review system performance and inform system improvements

Membership of the Committee comprises:

- Director of Trauma Services, The Royal Children's Hospital
- Director of Trauma Services, The Royal Melbourne Hospital
- Director of Trauma Services, Alfred Health
- General Manager, Ambulance Victoria
- Director, Adult Retrieval Victoria
- Director, Victorian Spinal Cord Service, Austin Health
- Senior Representative, Metropolitan Trauma Service

- Representative, Australasian College of Emergency Medicine
- Senior Representative, Regional Trauma Service
- Trauma Nurse, College of Emergency Nursing Australasia
- Chair, Victorian Trauma Committee, Royal Australasian College of Surgeons
- Representative, Transport Accident Commission
- Executive Representative, Epworth Rehabilitation
- Manager, Ambulance and Emergency Programs, Department of Health & Human Services

REFERENCES

1. Parliamentary Debates (Hansard) Forth-fifth Parliament, First session (1970–71). Legislative Council and Legislative Assembly. Victoria: Victorian Government Printer; 1970. p. 2801, 3-4.
2. Davison G. eMelbourne: The City Past and Present – Road Safety. 2014. http://www.emelbourne.net.au/biogs/EM01254b.htm (accessed June 4 2014).
3. McDermott F. Control of road trauma epidemic in Australia. *Ann R Coll Surg Engl* 1978; **60**(6): 437–50.
4. Clark B, Haworth N, Lenné M. The Victorian Parliamentary Road Safety Committee – A History of Inquiries and Outcomes Melbourne: Monash University Accident Research Centre, 2005.
5. Trinca GW. The Royal Australasian College of Surgeons and trauma care. *Aust N Z J Surg* 1995; **65**(6): 379–82.
6. Royal Australasian College of Surgeons. Trauma and Road Trauma Prevention. 2015. http://www.surgeons.org/member-services/interest-groups-sections/trauma/trauma-and-road-trauma-prevention/ (accessed March 26 2015).
7. Transport Accident Commission. Towards Zero 2016–2020 Strategy and Action Plan Victoria, Australia: Transport Accident Commission, 2016.
8. Dunn M. Rupert Murdoch, Keith Dunstan hailed as pioneers of journalism. Herald Sun. 2013 October 11, 2013.
9. Declare War on 1034: Let's end this grim harvest of tragedy. The Sun news-pictorial 1970 November 13; Sect. 1, 8.
10. DEATH. Where the young die good. The Sun news-pictorial 1970 November 17; Sect. 19.
11. Prior T. The princess who'll sleep forever. The Sun news-pictorial 1970 November 26; Sect. 3.
12. SAVED BY HER SEAT-BELT. The Sun news-pictorial 1970 December 29; Sect. 17.
13. Wilson B. 1034 lives – that means everyone...In Sea Lake, the town that is a symbol The Sun news-pictorial 1970 November 20; Sect. 28 – 9.
14. Some of us won't live. The Sun news-pictorial 1970 November 28; Sect. 1.
15. The Sun Psychologist. SO DEADLY – YOU? The Sun news-pictorial 1970 December 1; Sect. 8.
16. Catalogue of death...and file is closed. The Sun news-pictorial 1970 December 2; Sect. 34.
17. Don't be Mr 1034. The Sun news-pictorial 1970 December 15; Sect. 3.
18. Lad on push bike is victim. The Sun news-pictorial 1970 December 17; Sect. 1.
19. It's top danger day: Black Friday. The Sun news-pictorial 1970 December 18; Sect. 1.

20. Wilson B. WHEN DEATH IS A SECOND AWAY... The Sun news-pictorial 1970 December 18; Sect. 26 – 7.

21. Those danger hours! The Sun news-pictorial 1970 November 21; Sect. 1.

22. A truck driver – victim 976. The Sun news-pictorial 1970 November 19; Sect. 3.

23. Sanders R. Time to wake up, Mr Driver. The Sun news-pictorial 1970 November 21; Sect. 8.

24. Sinclair R. Drivers give the belt-up a miss. The Sun news-pictorial 1970 December 23; Sect. 11.

25. Parliamentary Debates (Hansard) Legislative Assembly, Fifty-sixth Parliament, First session: Tuesday, 7 August 2007 (Extract from book 11). Victoria: Victorian Government Printer; 2007. p. 2488–505.

26. Front page with sales figure. The Sun news-pictorial 1970 December 28; Sect. 1.

27. Baxendale R. Belt Up and Live road safety drive 'has lost passion'. The Australian. 2013 January 7, 2013.

28. Safety belt club. The Sun news-pictorial 1970 September 11; Sect. 15.

29. Commonwealth Department of Shipping and Transport, Road Safety Councils of Australia. Please Wear Your Seat Belt television commercial 1970. http://www.youtube.com/watch?v=Tc7_z4CH-iM (accessed July 26 2018).

30. Their own war on 1034. The Sun news-pictorial 1970 November 24; Sect. 1.

31. End this campaign? NOT ON YOUR LIFE. The Sun news-pictorial 1970 December 17; Sect. 8.

32. Joint Select Committee on Road Safety. Third Progress Report: Report upon an Investigation into the Desirability of the Compulsory Fitting and the Compulsory Wearing of Seat Belts. Victoria: Legislative Council, 1969.

33. Milne P. Fitting and Wearing of Seat Belts in Australia: The history of a successful countermeasure 1985.

34. Seat belt legislation. 2014. http://en.wikipedia.org/wiki/Seat_belt_legislation (accessed July 26 2018).

35. Fisher Jr F. Effectiveness of Safety Belt Usage Laws. Washington, USA: Peat, Marwick, Mitchell and Company, 1980.

36. AWARENESS 'CAN CHANGE LAWS'. The Sun news-pictorial 1970 November 14; Sect. 9.

37. Wilson B. Doctor: Why in hell won't they do it? The Sun news-pictorial 1970 November 16; Sect. 13.

38. 'Selfish Minority' is against safety. The Sun news-pictorial 1970 November 30; Sect. 17.

39. 'We have not done enough'. The Sun news-pictorial 1970 December 16; Sect. 36.

40. Safety-belt bill passes. The Sun news-pictorial 1970 December 3; Sect. 21.

41. Dixon D. SOBERING ODDS... The Sun news-pictorial 1970 December 19; Sect. 17.

42. Parliament of Victoria. About Parliament: On this day http://www.parliament.vic.gov.au/about/on-this-day?stask=decade&decade=1960 (accessed July 26 2018).

43. 56 people with a second chance. The Sun news-pictorial 1971 January 1; Sect. 1, 8.
44. McDermott F, Cordner S. Development of the Victorian State Trauma System: Clinical Perspective. Interview with Russell Gruen, Nathan Farrow and Andrew Silagy on June 6, 2013.
45. Figures tell the story... The Sun news-pictorial 1970 December 12; Sect. 1.
46. Trinca GW, Dooley BJ. The effects of seat belt legislation on road traffic injuries. *Aust N Z J Surg* 1977; **47**(2): 150–55.
47. McDermott FT, Hough DE. Reduction in road fatalities and injuries after legislation for compulsory wearing of seat belts: experience in Victoria and the rest of Australia. *The British journal of surgery* 1979; **66**(7): 518–21.
48. Trinca GW, Dooley BJ. The effects of mandatory seat belt wearing on the mortality and pattern of injury of car occupants involved in motor vehicle crashes in Victoria. *Med J Aust* 1975; **1**(22): 675–8.
49. More Drink tests urged (plus beer ad). The Sun news-pictorial 1970 December 23; Sect. 12.
50. McDermott F, Strang P. Compulsory blood alcohol testing of road crash casualties in Victoria: the first three years. *Med J Aust* 1978; **2**(14): 612–5.
51. Homel R. Crime on the Roads: Drinking and Driving. In: Vernon J, ed. Alcohol and Crime. Canberra: Australian Institute of Criminology; 1990: 67–82.
52. Hill R. Impaired Driving – A Message from Assistant Commissioner Robert Hill. Cops and Bloggers. Victoria: Victoria Police; 2013.
53. Homel R. Random breath testing in Australia: a complex deterrent. *Australian Drug and Alcohol Review* 1988; **7**: 231–41.
54. Moloney M. Random Breath Testing in the State of Victoria, Australia. 13th International Conference on Alcohol, Drugs and Traffic Safety (T'95). Adelaide, Australia 1995.
55. Transport Accident Commission. History of the TAC. 2014. http://www.tac. vic.gov.au/about-the-tac/our-organisation/what-we-do/history-of-the-tac (accessed July 26 2018).
56. Cockfield S. Road Safety – the Experience of the Transport Accident Commission in Victoria, Australia: Prepared for the Roundtable on Insurance Costs and Accident Risks (22–23 September 2011, Paris), 2011.
57. Elder RW, Shults RA, Sleet DA, et al. Effectiveness of mass media campaigns for reducing drinking and driving and alcohol-involved crashes: a systematic review. *American journal of preventive medicine* 2004; **27**(1): 57–65.
58. Transport Accident Commission. Drink Driving Case Study Victoria: Transport Accident Commission.
59. Transport Accident Commission. Girlfriend. 1989. http://www.youtube. com/watch?v=TfhR5w5uYWs (accessed July 26 2018).
60. Transport Accident Commission. Booze Bus. 1990. http://www.youtube. com/watch?v=J5_n5sgcbEc (accessed July 26 2018).
61. Transport Accident Commission. Joey. 1992. http://www.youtube.com/ watch?v=goDczc2KXtE (accessed July 26 2018).

62. Cameron M, Haworth N, Oxley J, Newstead S, Le T. Evaluation of Transport Accident Commission Road Safety Television Advertising. Melbourne: Monash University Accident Research Centre, 1993.

63. Newstead S, Cameron M, Gantzer S, Vulcan A. Modelling of some major factors influencing road trauma trends in Victoria 1989–93. Melbourne, Victoria: Monash University Accident Research Centre (MUARC), 1995.

64. Delaney A, Ward H, Cameron M. The History and Development of Speed Camera Use. Melbourne: Monash University Accident Research Centre, 2005.

65. Cameron M, Cavallo A, Gilbert A. Crash-based evaluation of the speed camera program in Victoria 1990–1991. Phase 1 : General effects. Phase 2: Effects of program mechanisms. Melbourne: Monash University Accident Research Centre, 1992.

66. Transport Accident Commission. June 7, 2014 2014. http://en.wikipedia.org/wiki/Transport_Accident_Commission (accessed July 27 2018).

67. Transport Accident Commission. Speed Cameras. 1990. http://www.youtube.com/watch?v=5hdekam-qNk (accessed July 26 2018).

68. Transport Accident Commission. Beach Road. 1990. http://www.youtube.com/watch?v=18jVzR86mCc (accessed July 26 2018).

69. Transport Accident Commission. Tracey. 1990. https://www.youtube.com/watch?v=JnUOCNw7Urs (accessed July 26 2018).

70. Transport Accident Commission. New road safety strategy – arrive alive 2008–2017. 2008. http://www.tac.vic.gov.au/about-the-tac/media-room/news-and-events/2008-media-releases/new-road-safety-strategy-arrive-alive-2008-2017 (accessed July 26 2018).

71. 2011–2012 Victorian Speed Limit Review Victoria: VicRoads, 2012.

72. Auditor General Victoria. Making travel safer: Victoria's speed enforcement program. Melbourne, Victoria, 2006.

73. Auditor General Victoria. Road Safety Camera Program: Victorian Auditor-General's Report August 2011. Melbourne, Victoria, 2011.

74. Cameras Save Lives. 2018. http://www.camerassavelives.vic.gov.au/ (accessed July 26 2018).

75. Hicks R. Mission: to upset, outrage and appal: 25 years of the TAC – and their 25 most powerful ads. 2012. http://mumbrella.com.au/mission-to-upset-outrage-and-appal-25-years-of-the-tac-and-their-25-most-powerful-ads-121326 (accessed July 26 2018).

76. Hennessy P. Reflections on TAC advertising: Interview with Peter Bragge, September 7 2015.

77. A course in road safety. . The Sunday Age August 20, 1995.

78. Transport Accident Commission. Bones. 1992. http://www.youtube.com/watch?v=O8gUXBvffdk (accessed July 26 2018).

79. Transport Accident Commission. The TAC Wipe Off 5 Campaign – A Case Study Victoria: Transport Accident Commission, 2002.

80. D'Elia A, Newstead S, Cameron M. Overall impact during 2001–2004 of Victorian speed-related package. Clayton, Victoria: Monash University Accident Research Centre, 2007.

81. Transport Accident Commission. Rename Speed. 2011. http://www.tac.vic.gov.au/road-safety/tac-campaigns/speed/rename-speed (accessed July 26 2018).

82. Donovan S. Welcome to the town of SpeedKills. 2011. http://www.abc.net.au/news/2011-02-18/welcome-to-the-town-of-speedkills/1948246 (accessed July 26 2018).

83. McDermott FT. Helmet efficacy in the prevention of bicyclist head injuries: Royal Australasian College of Surgeons initiatives in the introduction of compulsory safety helmet wearing in Victoria, Australia. *World J Surg* 1992; **16**(3): 379–83.

84. A history of road fatalities in Australia. In: Trewin D, ed. 2001: Year Book Australia ABS Catalogue No. 1301.0 ed. Canberra: Australian Bureau of Statistics 2001: 811–4.

85. Cameron MH, Vulcan AP, Finch CF, Newstead SV. Mandatory bicycle helmet use following a decade of helmet promotion in Victoria, Australia – an evaluation. *Accident; analysis and prevention* 1994; **26**(3): 325–37.

86. Cyclists Rights Action Group (CRAG). About Us. http://crag.asn.au/about (accessed July 26 2018).

87. Curnow WJ. The Cochrane Collaboration and bicycle helmets. *Accident; analysis and prevention* 2005; **37**(3): 569–73.

88. Robinson DL. Bicycle helmet legislation: can we reach a consensus? *Accident; analysis and prevention* 2007; **39**(1): 86–93.

89. Hooten KG, Murad GJ. Helmet Use and Cervical Spine Injury: A Review of Motorcycle, Moped, and Bicycle Accidents at a Level 1 Trauma Center. *J Neurotrauma* 2014.

90. Hagel BE, Barry Pless I. A critical examination of arguments against bicycle helmet use and legislation. *Accident; analysis and prevention* 2006; **38**(2): 277–8.

91. Attewell R, Glase K, McFadden M. Bicycle helmets and injury prevention: A formal review. Canberra: Australian Transport Safety Bureau, 2000.

92. Thompson DC, Rivara FP, Thompson R. Helmets for preventing head and facial injuries in bicyclists. *Cochrane database of systematic reviews (Online)* 1999; (2): CD001855.

93. McDermott F, Lane J. Protection afforded by cycle helmets. *Bmj* 1995; **310**(6987): 1138–9.

94. Victoria Police. Drug Driving in Victoria: Information provided for the Federal parliamentary inquiry into the effects of illicit drugs on families: Victoria Police, 2007.

95. Baldock M, Woolley J. Reviews of the effectiveness of random drug testing in Australia: The absence of crash-based evaluations. 2013 Australasian Road Safety Research, Policing & Education Conference; 2013 28th – 30th August; Brisbane, Queensland; 2013.

96. Random Roadside Drug Testing Program in Victoria: University of Queensland School of Population Health.

97. Lillebuen S. $40,000 fines loom for drunk, drugged drivers. The Age 2014.

REFERENCES

98. Road Safety Amendment Act 2014. Victoria, Australia; 2014. p. 9–17.

99. Transport Accident Commission. How safe is your car. 2018. http://www. howsafeisyourcar.com.au/ (accessed July 26 2018).

100. Dore J. Improving road safety: perspectives from Victoria's Transport Accident Commission. In: Lindquist E, Vincent S, Wanna J, eds. Delivering Policy Reform: Anchoring Significant Reforms in Turbulent Times. Canberra, Australia: ANU E Press; 2011.

101. Delaney A, Lough B, Whelan M, Cameron M. A Review Of Mass Media Campaigns in Road Safety. Melbourne: Monash University Accident Research Centre, 2004.

102. Transport Accident Commission. TACVictoria – YouTube channel. 2018. https://www.youtube.com/user/TACVictoria (accessed July 26 2018).

103. Yanovitsky I, Bennett C. Media Attention, Institutional Response, and Health Behavior Change: The Case of Drunk Driving, 1978–1996. *Communication Research* 1999; **26**(4): 429–53.

104. Bolitho J. John Bolitho interview with Peter Bragge and Russell Gruen 2014.

105. VicRoads. About VicRoads. December 12 2017. https://www.vicroads.vic. gov.au/about-vicroads (accessed July 26 2018).

106. VicRoads. Vehicle Registration & TAC fees December 11 2017. https:// www.vicroads.vic.gov.au/registration/registration-fees/vehicle-registration-fees (accessed July 26 2018).

107. Commission TA. Transport Accident Charges including GST and duty. 2018. http://www.tac.vic.gov.au/__data/assets/pdf_file/0020/270317/TAC-Charges-2018.pdf (accessed July 26 2018).

108. Cain J. Transport Accident Commission. Melbourne, 1992.

109. Parliament of Victoria. John William Galbally. http://www.parliament.vic. gov.au/re-member/details/1081-galbally-john-william (accessed July 26 2018).

110. Parliamentary Debates: Session 1950 – 51, Legislative Council and Legislative Assembly, August 21 – October 3, 1951. Victoria: J.J. Gourley, Government Printer; 1952. p. 4012–5.

111. Willmott N. 3rd PARTY MAY RISE: ROAD TOLL TO BLAME. The Sun news-pictorial 1970 December 17; Sect. 3.

112. Robinson M. Accident Compensation in Australia – No-fault schemes. Sydney: Legal Books Pty Ltd 1987.

113. Drabsch T. No Fault Compensation: Briefing Paper No 6/05. NSW, Australia: New South Wales Parliamentary Library; 2005.

114. Stylianou M. 'To strike a balance' A History of Victoria's Workers' Compensation Scheme, 1985–2010: Monash University Faculty of Arts / Institute for Safety, Compensation and Recovery Research 2011.

115. Parliamentary Debates (Hansard), Fiftieth Parliament, Spring Session 1986 Victoria: Victorian Government Printer; 1986. p. 164–50.

116. Eastman AB, Bishop GS, Walsh JC, Richardson JD, Rice CL. The economic status of trauma centers on the eve of health care reform. *J Trauma* 1994; **36**(6): 835–44; discussion 44–6.

117. Atkin C. Before the Victorian State Trauma System. NTRI conference. Melbourne; 2011.

118. Doyle R, Knowles R. Development of the Victorian State Trauma System: Political Perspective. Interview with Russell Gruen, Kate Martin and Susan Liew on August 31, 2012.

119. Fitzgerald M. The need for budgetry certainty NTRI conference. Melbourne; 2011.

120. Ranson D. What technique does the Coroner use and can we apply it to hospital deaths? Reviewing in-hospital mortality. Melbourne, Australia: Monash University Centre of Research Excellence in Patient Safety; 2010.

121. Nelson P. Pattern of Injury Survey of Automobile Accidents, Victoria, Australia, June 1971 – June 1973. Melbourne: Royal Australasian College of Surgeons Road Trauma Committee, 1974.

122. Trinca GW. Trauma and accident prevention: the role of the College. *Aust N Z J Surg* 1977; **47**(2): 133–4.

123. Royal Australasian College of Surgeons. Position Paper: Road Trauma Prevention Royal Australasian College of Surgeons 2013.

124. Atkin C, Freedman I, Rosenfeld JV, Fitzgerald M, Kossmann T. The evolution of an integrated State Trauma System in Victoria, Australia. *Injury* 2005; **36**(11): 1277–87.

125. Angwin B. Getting the right person to the right hospital at the right time: the role of the Metropolitan Fire Brigade. NTRI conference. Melbourne; 2011.

126. Silagy A. Using Death Information to Improve Trauma Care: A Study of Trauma Quality Improvement in Victoria, Australia [Minor Thesis]. Melbourne: Monash University 2013.

127. Danne P. Nurturing Change NTRI conference. Melbourne; 2011.

128. Gregory A. Blood, belts, booze and bikes: a history of the response of the Royal Australasian Colleg of Surgeons to the epidemic of road trauma. Melbourne, Australia: The Royal Australasian Colleg of Surgeons; 2008.

129. Cales RH, Trunkey DD. Preventable trauma deaths. A review of trauma care systems development. *JAMA* 1985; **254**(8): 1059–63.

130. Zollinger RW. Traffic injuries; a surgical problem. *AMA archives of surgery* 1955; **70**(5): 694–700.

131. Champion HR, Copes WS, Sacco WJ, et al. The Major Trauma Outcome Study: establishing national norms for trauma care. *J Trauma* 1990; **30**(11): 1356–65.

132. Death of Azaria Chamberlain. 2014. http://en.wikipedia.org/wiki/Death_of_Azaria_Chamberlain (accessed July 26 2018).

133. McDermott FT. The Consultative Committee on Road Traffic Fatalities in Victoria (1992–2006). NTRI conference. Melbourne; 2011.

134. Atkin C. Development of the Victorian State Trauma System. Interview with Andrew Silagy on September 25, 2013, 2013.

135. McDermott FT, Cordner SM, Tremayne AB. Evaluation of the medical management and preventability of death in 137 road traffic fatalities in

Victoria, Australia: an overview. Consultative Committee on Road Traffic Fatalities in Victoria. *J Trauma* 1996; **40**(4): 520–33; discussion 33–5.

136. State Government of Victoria Department of Health. Statutory Immunity: Frequently asked questions. Melbourne, Victoria: State Government of Victoria, 2013.

137. McDermott FT, Cordner SM, Tremayne AB. Consultative Committee on Road Traffic Fatalities: trauma audit methodology. *Aust N Z J Surg* 2000; **70**(10): 710–21.

138. McDermott F, Cordner S, Tremayne A. Report of the Consultative Committee on Road Traffic Fatalities in Victoria. Recommendations Advised by the Learned Colleges and Specialist Societies to Counter Problems Identified by the Consultative Committee in the Emergency and Clinical Management of Road Traffic Fatalities in Victoria. Melbourne, 1997.

139. McDermott FT, Cordner SM, Tremayne AB. Reproducibility of preventable death judgments and problem identification in 60 consecutive road trauma fatalities in Victoria, Australia. Consultative Committee on Road Traffic Fatalities in Victoria. *J Trauma* 1997; **43**(5): 831–9.

140. McDermott FT, Cordner SM, Tremayne AB, Consultative Committee on Road traffic F. Road traffic fatalities in Victoria, Australia and changes to the trauma care system. *The British journal of surgery* 2001; **88**(8): 1099–104.

141. McDermott FT, Cordner SM, Tremayne AB. Management deficiencies and death preventability in 120 Victorian road fatalities (1993–1994). The Consultative Committee on Road Traffic Fatalities in Victoria. *Aust N Z J Surg* 1997; **67**(9): 611–8.

142. McDermott FT, Cooper GJ, Hogan PL, Cordner SM, Tremayne AB. Evaluation of the prehospital management of road traffic fatalities in Victoria, Australia. *Prehospital and disaster medicine* 2005; **20**(4): 219–27.

143. Danne P, Brazenor G, Cade R, et al. The major trauma management study: an analysis of the efficacy of current trauma care. *Aust N Z J Surg* 1998; **68**(1): 50–7.

144. Cooper DJ, McDermott FT, Cordner SM, Tremayne AB. Quality assessment of the management of road traffic fatalities at a level I trauma center compared with other hospitals in Victoria, Australia. Consultative Committee on Road Traffic Fatalities in Victoria. *J Trauma* 1998; **45**(4): 772–9.

145. Davies JA. Patients die after errors at hospitals. The Sunday Age. July 29 1995.

146. Mock C, Juillard C, Brundage B, Goosen J, Joshipura M, (eds). Guidelines for trauma quality improvement programmes. Geneva: World Health Organization; 2009.

147. Brook C. Policy development for the Victorian State Trauma System. NTRI conference. Melbourne; 2011.

148. Mullins RJ. A historical perspective of trauma system development in the United States. *J Trauma* 1999; **47**(3 Suppl): S8–14.

149. Gruen RL, Pitt V, Green S, Parkhill A, Campbell D, Jolley D. The effect of provider case volume on cancer mortality: systematic review and meta-analysis. *CA Cancer J Clin* 2009; **59**(3): 192–211.

150. Review of Trauma and Emergency Services Victoria 1999: Report of the Ministerial Taskforce on Trauma and Emergency Services and the Department of Human Services Working Party on Emergency and Trauma Services. Melbourne 1999.
151. Kennedy M. The process of change. NTRI conference. Melbourne; 2011.
152. National Road Trauma Advisory Council. Report of the Working Party on Trauma Systems, 1993.
153. Finkel E. Australian metropolitan health-care services plan. *The Lancet* 1996; **348**(9035, October 1996): 1163.
154. Civil I. Focus on trauma systems/centres: an Australasian perspective. 1999; **1**: 193–7.
155. Judson R. The Role of the Victorian State Trauma Outcomes Registry NTRI conference. Melbourne; 2011.
156. Bennett S, Newman G. Victorian Election 1999 – Research Paper no. 19, 1999–2000: Department of the Parliamentary Library, Information and Research Services 2010.
157. Thwaites J. Political perspective on the VSTS: the politics of change. NTRI conference. Melbourne; 2011.
158. Standen P. The impact of the Victorian State Trauma System on rural communities. NTRI conference. Melbourne; 2011.
159. Trauma towards 2014: Review and future directions of the Victorian State Trauma System. Victoria: State of Victoria, Department of Human Services, 2009.
160. Victorian State Trauma Outcome Registry and Monitoring Group. Victorian State Trauma Registry 1 July 2009 to 30 June 2010: Summary report. Melbourne, 2011.
161. Gabbe BJ, Simpson PM, Sutherland AM, et al. Improved functional outcomes for major trauma patients in a regionalized, inclusive trauma system. *Ann Surg* 2012; **255**(6): 1009–15.
162. Victorian State Trauma Outcome Registry and Monitoring Group. Victorian State Trauma Registry 1 July 2010 to 30 June 2011: Summary report. Melbourne, 2012.
163. Gabbe BJ, Lyons RA, Fitzgerald MC, Judson R, Richardson J, Cameron PA. Reduced Population Burden of Road Transport-Related Major Trauma After Introduction of an Inclusive Trauma System. *Ann Surg* 2014.
164. Gabbe BJ, Biostat GD, Lecky FE, et al. The effect of an organized trauma system on mortality in major trauma involving serious head injury: a comparison of the United kingdom and victoria, australia. *Ann Surg* 2011; **253**(1): 138–43.
165. Gabbe BJ, Lyons RA, Lecky FE, et al. Comparison of mortality following hospitalisation for isolated head injury in England and Wales, and Victoria, Australia. *PLoS One* 2011; **6**(5): e20545.
166. Willett K. A new trauma system for the United Kingdom. NTRI conference. Melbourne; 2011.

167. Gruen RL, Gabbe BJ, Stelfox HT, Cameron PA. Indicators of the quality of trauma care and the performance of trauma systems. *The British journal of surgery* 2012; **99 Suppl 1**: 97–104.

168. Ambulance Victoria. 2015 – 2016 Annual Report. Melbourne, Victoria, 2016.

169. Trauma Victoria. Pre-hospital triage guideline: Version 1.0. Melbourne, Victori, 2014.

170. Definition of triage. 2017. https://en.oxforddictionaries.com/definition/triage (accessed July 27 2018).

171. Kennedy M. Getting the right patient to the right hospital at the right time: the role of Adult Retrieval Victoria. NTRI conference. Melbourne; 2011.

172. Evans C. Adult Retrieval Victoria – A Trauma Snapshot. NTRI conference. Melbourne; 2011.

173. Ambulance Historical Society of Victoria. History. 2017. http://www.ahsv. org.au/history/ (accessed July 27 2018).

174. Bernard SA, Nguyen V, Cameron P, et al. Prehospital rapid sequence intubation improves functional outcome for patients with severe traumatic brain injury: a randomized controlled trial. *Ann Surg* 2010; **252**(6): 959–65.

175. Fitzgerald M, Cameron P, Mackenzie C, et al. Trauma resuscitation errors and computer-assisted decision support. *Arch Surg* 2011; **146**(2): 218–25.

176. Khan F, Baguley IJ, Cameron ID. 4: Rehabilitation after traumatic brain injury. *The Medical journal of Australia* 2003; **178**(6): 290–5.

177. Peter Cameron profile interview with Peter Bragge and Melissa Marino, December 2 2016.

178. Monash University: Victorian State Trauma Outcome Registry and Monitoring Group. Victorian State Trauma Registry 1 July 2012 to 30 June 2013: Summary report. Melbourne: Victorian State Trauma Registry, 2014.

179. Victorian Government Department of Health. State Trauma Committee: Terms of Reference and Composition, 2013.

180. Cameron PA, Gabbe BJ, McNeil JJ, et al. The trauma registry as a statewide quality improvement tool. *J Trauma* 2005; **59**(6): 1469–76.

181. Cameron PA, Gabbe BJ, Cooper DJ, Walker T, Judson R, McNeil J. A statewide system of trauma care in Victoria: effect on patient survival. *Med J Aust* 2008; **189**(10): 546–50.

182. McDermott FT, Cordner SM, Cooper DJ, Winship VC, Consultative Committee on Road Traffic Fatalities in V. Management deficiencies and death preventability of road traffic fatalities before and after a new trauma care system in Victoria, Australia. *J Trauma* 2007; **63**(2): 331–8.

183. Ivers NM, Grimshaw JM, Jamtvedt G, et al. Growing literature, stagnant science? Systematic review, meta-regression and cumulative analysis of audit and feedback interventions in health care. *J Gen Intern Med* 2014; **29**(11): 1534–41.

184. Grimshaw JM, Eccles MP, Lavis JN, Hill SJ, Squires JE. Knowledge translation of research findings. *Implementation science : IS* 2012; **7**(1): 50.

185. Allsopp C. Trauma Program Manager's Role in Quality Improvement. NTRI conference. Melbourne; 2011.
186. Cameron P. Using Data to Drive System Change. NTRI conference. Melbourne; 2011.
187. Newstead S, Delaney A, Watson L, Cameron M. A model for considering the 'total safety' of the light passenger vehicle fleet. Report No. 228 August 2004. Melbourne, Victoria: Monash University Accident Research Centre (MUARC), 2004.
188. Kennedy MP, Gabbe BJ, McKenzie BA. Impact of the introduction of an integrated adult retrieval service on major trauma outcomes. *Emerg Med J* 2015; **32**(11): 833–9.
189. Brennan PW, Everest ER, Griggs WM, et al. Risk of death among cases attending South Australian major trauma services after severe trauma: the first 4 years of operation of a state trauma system. *J Trauma* 2002; **53**(2): 333–9.
190. Nathens AB, Jurkovich GJ, Cummings P, Rivara FP, Maier RV. The effect of organized systems of trauma care on motor vehicle crash mortality. *JAMA* 2000; **283**(15): 1990–4.
191. Victorian State Trauma Outcome Registry and Monitoring Group. Victorian State Trauma System and Registry Annual Report, 1 July 2015 to 30 June 2016. Melbourne, 2017.
192. Access Economics. The economic cost of spinal cord injury and traumatic brain injury in Australia. Report by Access Economics Pty Limited for The Victorian Neurotrauma Initiative. 2009: 115 pages.
193. Institute for Safety Compensation and Recovery Research. Neurotrauma Research Strategy 2011–2015. Melbourne: Institute for Safety, Compensation and Recovery Research, 2012.
194. Cromarty F. Achieving Independence NTRI conference. Melbourne; 2011.
195. Gruen RL, Elliott JH, Nolan ML, et al. Sustainability science: an integrated approach for health-programme planning. *Lancet* 2008; **372**(9649): 1579–89.
196. Mock C, Lormand J, Goosen J, Joshipura M, Peden M. Guidelines for essential trauma care. Geneva: World Health Organization, 2004.
197. Parliament of Victoria. Committees; 57th Parliament; Road Safety; Inquiries. 2017. https://www.parliament.vic.gov.au/57th-parliament/rsc/inquiries?showyear=0&section_id=471&cat_id=453 (accessed July 27 2018).
198. McDermott F, Cordner S, Winship V. Addressing inadequacies in Victoria's trauma system: responses of the Consultative Committee on Road Traffic Fatalities and Victorian trauma services. *Emerg Med Australas* 2010; **22**(3): 224–31.

INDEX

(Note: Page numbers followed by *i* indicate illustration)

CPSIA information can be obtained
at www.ICGtesting.com
Printed in the USA
BVHW042324231118
533688BV00003B/31/P